COPING WITH COELIAC DISEASE

KAREN BRODY is a freelance writer who writes mostly on
health issues. She has been a student at the Natural Gourmet
Cookery School in New York, where she studied the
relationship between food and healing and how to cook for
special diets.

Overcoming Common Problems Series

For a full list of titles please contact
Sheldon Press, Marylebone Road, London NW1 4DU

The Assertiveness Workbook
A plan for busy women
JOANNA GUTMANN

Beating the Comfort Trap
DR WINDY DRYDEN AND JACK
GORDON

Birth Over Thirty Five
SHEILA KITZINGER

Body Language
How to read others' thoughts by their
gestures
ALLAN PEASE

Body Language in Relationships
DAVID COHEN

Calm Down
How to cope with frustration and anger
DR PAUL HAUCK

Cancer – A Family Affair
NEVILLE SHONE

The Candida Diet Book
KAREN BRODY

Caring for Your Elderly Parent
JULIA BURTON-JONES

Comfort for Depression
JANET HORWOOD

Coping Successfully with Hayfever
DR ROBERT YOUNGSON

Coping Successfully with Migraine
SUE DYSON

Coping Successfully with Pain
NEVILLE SHONE

Coping Successfully with PMS
KAREN EVENNETT

Coping Successfully with Panic Attacks
SHIRLEY TRICKETT

**Coping Successfully with Prostate
Problems**
ROSY REYNOLDS

**Coping Successfully with Irritable
Bladder**
JENNIFER HUNT

**Coping Successfully with Your Irritable
Bowel**
ROSEMARY NICOL

**Coping Successfully with Joint
Replacement**
DR TOM SMITH

Coping with Anxiety and Depression
SHIRLEY TRICKETT

Coping with Blushing
DR ROBERT EDELMANN

Coping with Breast Cancer
DR EADIE HEYDERMAN

Coping with Bronchitis and Emphysema
DR TOM SMITH

Coping with Candida
SHIRLEY TRICKETT

Coping with Chronic Fatigue
TRUDIE CHALDER

Coping with Cystitis
CAROLINE CLAYTON

Coping with Depression and Elation
DR PATRICK McKEON

Coping with Eczema
DR ROBERT YOUNGSON

Coping with Endometriosis
JO MEARS

Coping with Psoriasis
PROFESSOR RONALD MARKS

Coping with Schizophrenia
DR STEVEN JONES AND DR FRANK
TALLIS

Coping with Stomach Ulcers
DR TOM SMITH

Coping with Thyroid Problems
DR JOAN GOMEZ

Coping with Thrush
CAROLINE CLAYTON

Coping with Your Cervical Smear
KAREN EVENNETT

Crunch Points for Couples
JULIA COLE

Curing Arthritis Exercise Book
MARGARET HILLS AND JANET
HORWOOD

Overcoming Common Problems Series

Overcoming Common Problems Series

Overcoming Common Problems

Coping with Coeliac Disease

Karen Brody

sheldon**PRESS**

First published in Great Britain in 1997
Sheldon Press, SPCK, Holy Trinity Church, Marylebone Road, London NW1 4DU

British Library Cataloguing-in-Publication Data
A catalogue for this book is available from the British Library

ISBN 0–85969–768–1

Photoset by Deltatype Limited, Birkenhead, Merseyside
Printed in Great Britain by
Biddles Ltd, Guildford and King's Lynn

Contents

For Kathleen Ogborn, a very special, caring woman who went through many years of her life as an undiagnosed coeliac. This book is dedicated to her memory.

Acknowledgements

Somehow, despite constant powercuts throughout Nairobi, I wrote this book. I'd therefore like to acknowledge the Nakumatt/Ukay generator, for all the background noise it provided while writing this book. Also the Kenya Power and Electricity Company as its schedule for powercuts was never correct, but it came through in the end, providing me with enough power to finish the manuscript without having to purchase an expensive electrical device.

Special thanks to Donna Ambury, for our lively conversations on coeliac disease, food and healing. May you continue to have good health and derive strength from your new eating habits. Your words provided me with much food for thought.

Warm thanks to my Father-in-law James, for your cheerful assistance with ideas and news about coeliac disease.

Thanks to my Mom, for being a super mom throughout the years, and always being open-minded about accepting different eating habits.

And to Tim, who puts up with me, and nurtures my ideas at the dinner table.

Introduction

You as the patient are in charge of your own body. The physician and his staff, your family and friends serve as helpers, consultants. Never forget that you must take an active interest in your bodily welfare.

Lloyd Rosenvold, MD, *Can a Gluten-free Diet Help? How?*

This book could change your life. Not because it's well written or provides all the right information for you, but because you – or someone who cares about you – took the step to buy a book on how to cope with your coeliac condition. Taking this step will change your life.

Buying a book on coping does not mean you are not coping or that all the coeliacs you will read about in this book cope with the disease in the same way you do. On the contrary, coping means you're taking care of yourself, empowering yourself with information that may help you on those days when you feel rotten, experience a set-back and need some reassurance that you will feel better once again.

You will quickly discover in this book that all coeliacs cope differently with their condition. This is true for most physical ailments, and especially when the treatment is food-related. So why write a book about coping? Because all personal experiences have meaning, whether they are suitable for you or not. Reading about how others cope can often spark new ideas that you never thought of. Think of all the different coping strategies you'll read about in this book like something to dip into, taking what you like and discarding the rest. No strategy is right or wrong; each coeliac is an expert, with knowledge of how to cope. This book will help you build on your knowledge.

Coeliac disease is a very serious disease if untreated, so you must stick strictly to a gluten-free diet in order to feel better. This may seem difficult at times. For example, food manufacturers often do not accurately label their products with the exact ingredients they contain or suddenly change their ingredients without relabelling the product for several months. Scenarios like this can make a coeliac go bonkers. 'Can I eat it or can't I?', that really is the question for most coeliacs. Hopefully this book will reassure you that you are not alone. There are many coeliacs asking the same questions out there, in countries all around the world.

This book has been written to give you answers about coeliac disease now, bearing in mind that the medical knowledge about coeliac disease changes and the advice coeliacs will get from individual doctors may differ. As a coeliac, you must devise your own plan to cope with coeliac disease, while always keeping yourself up to date on the current medical research and findings. Research on coeliac disease may be changing every day, but the goal of every coeliac is similar: to feel better now. People's health cannot wait for research. If you know you are a coeliac, the key to feeling better is to stick strictly to a gluten-free diet.

If you are reading this book and think you or someone you know may have coeliac disease, consult your doctor and explain your symptoms and how they relate to coeliac disease. As the symptoms of coeliac disease mimic those of many other conditions, you cannot be sure you have coeliac disease without having tests. These can be done by referral from your GP. There are many undiagnosed coeliacs, feeling awful and not aware that eating a gluten-free diet could be their ticket to better health. It would not be wise to start a gluten-free diet before having the tests, though, because this can often spoil the accuracy of the results. So have the tests first – never self-diagnose.

Coping is a way of healing. You can never be cured of coeliac disease, but you can live a completely healthy life if you follow a gluten-free diet. As one coeliac told me:

> after I adjusted to the gluten-free diet I began to feel better because I began to accept the gluten-free diet and just get on with things instead of brooding about having coeliac disease and being on this special diet. I now take my gluten-free snacks with me, so I'm always prepared and never without food. I think it's this kind of attitude that has made me feel so much better.

This book will give you strategies for coping on the diet. Try some and see if they work for you. Your health depends on adhering to this diet; it will change your life.

1

How to find out whether or not you have coeliac disease

A challenging diagnosis

Mary

Mary, 29, had felt severely fatigued for years, but considered this to be due to her hectic schedule of long hours in the office and taking care of her bedridden mother most weekends. In general, though, she felt very healthy and had no other physical ailments. Her doctor encouraged her to be tested for anaemia, to see if this condition was causing her fatigue. The test results were positive, so Mary immediately began to recieve iron injections to treat the anaemia. About a year later, still feeling fatigued, Mary went back to her doctor and they discussed what else might be causing this. Two years later, after many frustrating appointments with consultants, Mary had her answer – she had coeliac disease.

Thomas

Thomas, 4, never thrived as a baby. Despite all the food his parents fed him, he could not gain weight and his stomach was bloated. Thomas' pediatrician immediately suspected coeliac disease. The results were positive.

Sue

Sue, 65, had experienced gastrointestinal (GI) problems virtually her entire life. She had had recurring anaemia since she was 16, and experienced periodic bouts of diarrhoea that made it difficult to go about her daily life. In her 40s, the GI pains worsened, often feeling like someone was stabbing her in the stomach, and the periods of diarrhoea lasted longer and longer each time. She had always been embarrassed by her excessive gas, but now the gas seemed uncontrollable. She often felt 'spaced out' and began losing weight rapidly. Many trips to doctors produced no definitive answers. Sue was withering away and, as a result, became severely depressed, assuming she was going to die. Then, one day, Sue's husband returned home and said someone at his office had coeliac disease and thought Sue should go for tests to see if this might be the cause of her problems. She was tested, and it was confirmed that she did have coeliac disease.

Coeliac (pronounced 'seeleeack') disease is very difficult to diagnose. Virtually no two coeliacs have the same case history, as we have just seen. There are typical coeliac symptoms, but many coeliacs also demonstrate atypical symptoms. This is the challenge that doctors face when they are confronted with common complaints like fatigue, stomach pains and diarrhoea. These types of symptoms can point to hundreds of different conditions, some not very serious and others that may be life-threatening. Doctors often have to put together a large puzzle of various symptoms before they decide to carry out tests to see if you have coeliac disease. Both the patient and doctor (especially with adult cases of coeliac disease) are often equally frustrated in their search for a definitive diagnosis. In the case of older people, the road before they're diagnosed with coeliac disease is often longer than most because doctors rarely think of coeliac disease instantly as older people are prone to an array of health problems anyway.

This chapter is designed to give you a better understanding of the typical symptoms coeliacs suffer. Every coeliac will not necessarily have these 'typical' symptoms, however. As the spectrum of symptoms for coeliac disease is wide-ranging, it can be confusing and self-defeating for you to self-diagnose.

You may have already been diagnosed as having coeliac disease by your doctor, so know for sure that you have it. If you haven't been diagnosed but suspect you have coeliac disease, make your doctor aware of your concerns. Not everyone who has the typical symptoms has coeliac disease. In fact, some people with coeliac disease have very few symptoms, while others, who have all the typical symptoms, don't have coeliac disease! So, never presume you have coeliac disease, go to a specialist for the tests.

Physical symptoms

Most coeliacs never feel well. Those with severe symptoms might not be able to make it to work on a daily basis or shy away from social activities because it would take them away from the lavatory, which becomes like a second home. Even coeliacs who claim to 'feel fine' often experience a lower quality of life than they could have – they just don't know that they could feel a lot better. Only after going on a gluten-free diet do they realize that their body can perform at a much higher capacity than it has been doing.

As there is no 'typical' coeliac, the following list should be read with the understanding that these are the most common physical symptoms coeliacs exhibit, but that there are extremes at both ends of the spectrum.

Common symptoms in adults

- Diarrhoea.
- Bloating and abdominal distension.
- Abdominal pain.
- Excessive flatulence.
- Nausea, vomiting.
- Passing fatty stools that float rather than sink (steatorrhoea).
- Constipation.
- Fatigue.
- Iron deficiency.
- Chronic fatigue.
- Weight loss.
- Lactose intolerance (intolerance of dairy products).
- Bone pain, muscle weakness.
- Depression.

Common symptoms in children

- Failure to thrive.
- Small stature.
- Abdominal distension, with or without pain.
- Stool abnormalities.
- Frequent diarrhoea.
- Vomiting.
- Nutritional deficiencies.
- Mood abnormalities, irritability.
- Inability to concentrate.

These symptoms of coeliac disease occur because a coeliac's small intestine is not able to absorb nutrients normally (this is explained in more detail in Chapter 2). It is thought that coeliacs experience such a wide variety of symptoms because the amount of intestinal damage in each individual is different, and the more intestinal damage, the more severe the symptoms.

While some of the symptoms of coeliac disease resemble those of irritable bowel syndrome (IBS), coeliacs do not have IBS. Irritable bowel syndrome occurs in the lower bowel and is not associated with anaemia and weight loss, whereas coeliac disease is. A person with IBS may be sensitive to gluten, but this is not an immune system response (whereas it is in coeliac disease), it is a neurohormonal response. Not all gluten-induced bowel disorders are due to coeliac disease, but it does happen that some people are incorrectly diagnosed as having IBS when they actually have coeliac disease, colitis or Crohn's disease.

Psychological symptoms also tend to appear in both adults and children with coeliac disease. It is common for undiagnosed adult coeliacs to experience bouts of depression, often due to their constant physical suffering and, sometimes, a lack of understanding on the part of family and friends. Coeliac children can also exhibit mood disorders, like acting up at school or general irritability. Of course, depression and mood disorders can be experienced by almost anyone, but if they are combined with some of the physical symptoms above, you should ask your doctor to check whether or not this is because of coeliac disease. If a gluten-free diet is all it will take to get rid of the psychological distress then it's worth making the trip to the doctor.

You may now be thinking, 'I have diarrhoea, chronic fatigue, depression and abdominal pain, maybe I have coeliac disease'. Maybe, but these four symptoms are also typical of other diseases, like giardia and Crohn's disease. So, don't get into 'maybes' and 'could bes', go to your doctor and find out for sure.

Diagnosing your condition

First, relax. If you do have coeliac disease you are lucky – the prescription involves no drugs, just dietary changes. Before you are declared a coelic, there are three steps you must take:

- see your doctor
- have a small intestinal biopsy
- test your response to a gluten-free diet.

Going to see your doctor

Start with a visit to your doctor. Many coeliacs have already been to their doctor so many times their head is spinning, so it may seem like a waste of time to you. It's not. Your doctor is able to refer you to a gastroenterologist who specializes in coeliac disease.

Such a specialist will take great care to review your case. They will begin by asking you to tell them your medical history. Important considerations include your physical symptoms, such as diarrhoea, bloating, the colour and form of your stools, any weight fluctuations and if you have any family members who have been diagnosed as having coeliac disease or who have experienced symptoms similar to yours. This is your chance to tell the specialist every relevant medical fact about yourself. If you think you may forget something, don't be shy, write yourself notes on a piece of paper and take them with you to the appointment. The specialist wants you to remember everything because it will help them make a more informed diagnosis.

You will probably also be given a physical examination. This is when the specialist will check for signs of pallor (due to anaemia), emaciation, hypotension (low blood pressure), skin lesions, bruising easily (due to lack of vitamin K), a protruding and distended abdomen and any severe vitamin deficiencies, like muscle spasms due to magnesium and/or calcium deficiency. Your specific symptoms will determine what the specialist checks, so don't be concerned if everything just mentioned is not checked or if additional areas are examined.

Some specialists will perform laboratory tests – to determine malabsorption syndromes – to help them diagnose whether or not you have coeliac disease. These tests could include various blood tests to check for nutritional anaemia, electrolytes, protein, calcium and serum carotene; stool examinations to check the weight of your stool or for the presence of greater than normal levels of fat; immunological tests to check for gliadin antibodies and other relevant antibodies.

If the specialist is convinced that you demonstrate impairment of the lining of your small intestine, the next step is to perform a small intestinal biopsy.

Having a small intestinal biopsy

The only way to know definitely whether or not you have coeliac disease is to have a small intestinal biopsy (also called an endoscopy or jejunal biopsy) done and, if the results of this are positive, how you react to a gluten-free diet will confirm the diagnosis. The biopsy will determine whether the lining of the small intestine, the mucosa, is damaged or not.

To have the biopsy done, you will need to go to hospital as a day patient. The actual procedure takes approximately 10–15 minutes,

7

but expect to spend at least the full morning or afternoon in hospital because normally you will be given a local anaesthetic. Make sure someone can pick you up and stay with you for a while afterwards because the anaesthetic often makes people drowsy. Otherwise, there are no side-effects to this simple surgical procedure.

The procedure itself involves a narrow flexible tube being passed down your throat, through the stomach and into the upper small intestine. A fine cylinder with a hole and a knife device are at the end of the tube. Using suction through the tube, a small piece of the intestinal lining is taken into the hole and the knife then cuts it off and closes the hole. The tissue sample is then taken out and inspected under a microscope.

The difference between normal bowel tissue and that found in a coeliac is often remarkable. Chapter 2 explains this in more detail, and there you will see diagrams that show just how annihilated the absorptive surface of a coeliac's small intestine can be.

Can there be a false negative test? Yes, it does happen, but not often. If the surgeon took the biopsy from the wrong area or if you began a gluten-free diet on your own before the biopsy, these two factors could affect the results. Otherwise, most biopsy results are accurate.

Testing your response to a gluten-free diet

If your biopsy is positive, you will be put on a gluten-free diet immediately and most specialists will monitor what improvement you experience for at least the first six months after you start the diet. Many coeliacs begin to see an improvement in their physical health within days of starting the diet. After six months, depending on how bad you were feeling before, you should feel dramatically better. This period is considered the 'test' phase because if you are not getting better, the specialist will question the diagnosis. If you strictly adhere to a gluten-free diet – with no cheating – you should not feel bad after you have been on the diet for a while. If you do, you may not have coeliac disease or you may have lingering food intolerances. You and your doctor need to look further into this in order to make an accurate diagnosis.

As mentioned above, do not begin a gluten-free diet before you have a biopsy because it can alter the results of the test. You may be tempted to 'just try' a gluten-free diet and find you feel a lot better, but this does not necessarily mean you have coeliac disease. Many people – especially those who have bowel problems or an intolerance of gluten – feel better for a while on a gluten-free diet but they are not coeliacs. So, see your doctor and have a biopsy before you start the diet.

Treatment

'No bread!', Michael shouted as his doctor handed him a list of foods to avoid on a gluten-free diet. His face dropped. 'It's just not possible! I want a pill. Give me any pill!'

The doctor moved to the other end of the room, fearing Michael might snap at any moment. 'No Michael,' the doctor said, 'there is no medicine that can help you. The only answer is to change your diet.'

'You must be joking. What am I going to eat?' Michael lowered his head and slouched deep down into his chair.

Change your diet and you will feel better. This is the advice everyone recieves when they are diagnosed as having coeliac disease. The key to good health if you have this disease is to change your diet. You could try to pop every pill imaginable, but it would do no good. You need to adhere strictly to a gluten-free diet for life because coeliac disease is incurable. Some children are sensitive to gluten at an early age and grow out of it; they do not have coeliac disease. Once a coelic, always a coeliac. Some coeliac children, after they have gone on a gluten-free diet for a while, can go through a period of 'feeling well' while eating gluten, but the lining of their small intestine is still being damaged and they will often begin to feel poorly in later years.

When gluten is eliminated from your diet, the small intestine is often able to repair itself completely, but you will still always have the potential to damage the lining of your intestine if you eat gluten. That is why even eating just a little food that has gluten in it once in a while could have disastrous effects on a coeliac, as the small intestine could quickly return to its damaged state and all your symptoms could recur.

The challenge for every coeliac is to start and stay on a gluten-free diet. Western diets contain lots of foods with gluten in them – wheat, oats, barley, rye and their derivatives – so every coeliac must educate themselves with up-to-date dietary information on gluten-free foods (see Chapter 5 for more details). It may appear overwhelming in the beginning when you seem to be cutting out all the foods you've lived on most of your life, but it does get easier. Lots of coeliacs are coping on this diet and, in fact, enjoying a more varied diet than ever before.

While a gluten-free diet is the primary treatment for all coeliacs, some coeliacs find that even after they go on a gluten-free diet they still have some physical symptoms and need to look further into it. The cause of these lingering physical symptoms can range from additional food sensitivities (common food sensitivities are those to lactose, corn, caffeine, citrus fruits) to systemic yeast infections (candida). As coeliacs have usually been sick for some time, their immune systems are weak and the body often needs a readjustment period, the length of which depends on the individual. Older people will often take longer to recover because, if they have had coeliac disease, undiagnosed, for a long time, their immune system will be weak.

Often lactose intolerance can continue to cause bowel problems for a short period after going on a gluten-free diet, so you may want to eliminate foods that contain lactose first. Then try eliminating other foods if that doesn't clear up your symptoms. Soon your small intestine should recover and you should be able to eat anything except gluten. It is important to consult your doctor in all this to consider your particular case because for every coeliac the extent of the damage to their small intestine, their symptoms and needs are different.

It may seem radical to change your diet, yet the fact that this treatment is safe, effective and has no side-effects should be welcomed, not greeted with horror. If you take going on a gluten-free diet seriously, you will feel better. If you don't take it seriously, you could run the risk of having more medical problems in the future. It's your choice.

2

What is coeliac disease?

A historical perspective

The first mention of coeliac disease was by Arataeus of Cappadocia, a contemporary of the Roman physician Galen, in AD 250. His description of childhood and adult coeliac disease showed a remarkable understanding of it. The text was edited and translated from the Greek for the Sydenham Society of England in 1856.

The next documented account of coeliac disease was by Samuel Gee at St Bartholomew's Hospital in London in 1888. He indicated that, 'to regulate the food is the main part of the treatment. ... The allowance of farinaceous foods must be small ... but if the patient can be cured at all, it must be by means of diet'. This widely quoted description of his findings added significantly to the medical profession's understanding of the cause of coeliac disease and increased clinical interest.

In 1908, a paediatrican named Herter wrote a book on coeliac children. Herter was considered such an authority on this subject that the condition was often known as Gee-Herter's disease. He is best known for contributing the idea that 'fats are better tolerated than carbohydrates'. This idea was supported and built on in 1918 by another paediatrician, Sir Frederick Still, who noted the harmful effects of bread in coeliac disease. 'Unfortunately, one form of starch that seems particularly liable to aggravate the symptoms is bread. I know of no adequate substitute'.

Howland, in 1921, developed these ideas further in an address he gave to the American Pediatric Society entitled *Prolonged Intolerance to Carbohydrates*. His three-stage diet – typically referred to as the milk/protein diet – allowed carbohydrates only in the last stage and then they had to be added 'very gradually with the most careful observation of the digestive capacity'.

A few years later, Hass advocated the banana diet, which was essentially low in carbohydrates, except for bananas. By 1938, Hass published his finding that a minute quantity of foods containing carbohydrates will produce fatty diarrhoea in someone with coeliac disease even when they are taking hardly any fat in the diet, but when they follow a high-carbohydrate diet – in the form of bananas – this will be well-tolerated, even though a greater amount of fat is being eaten.

A Dutch paediatrician named Dicke made the next giant leap forward in the treatment of coeliac disease by suggesting in his 1950 doctoral thesis from the University of Utrecht that certain dietary grains were harmful to children. He was able to show that coeliac children improved dramatically when wheat, rye and oat flours were excluded from their diet. He pointed out that during the war years, coeliac children in Holland greatly improved when grain products were in short supply. Throughout the rest of Europe, where children were regularly eating grains, coeliac children's health had not improved. Then, after the War, when grains began flowing into Holland again, coeliac children started to feel bad again. Dicke's observations formed the basis of the treatment of coeliacs thereafter – the gluten-free diet.

Progress in solving the mysteries of coeliac disease began to take off after Dicke's observations. The first accurate description of an abnormality in the lining of a coeliac's small intestine was provided in 1954 by Dr Paulley, a physician in Ipswich. This became the most noteworthy feature on which doctors could then base a diagnosis of coeliac disease. While it was noted that this abnormality was an inflammation, the exact nature of this is still being investigated. Two years later, Margot Shiner developed a small bowel biopsy tube which became the standard method of diagnosing the condition. And two years after that, in 1958, Cyrus Rubin and his colleagues demonstrated that childhood and adult coeliac disease were identical diseases, with the same clinical and pathological features.

Since these breakthroughs in the understanding of coeliac disease, there have been numerous physicians who have contributed to research on the disease, building on the strides forward made in the past. Like all research, some hypotheses contradict others, so you may come across slight variations in the recommendations you are given for treatment using a gluten-free diet. History has brought us very far, but the challenge is always to know more. The more we know about coeliac disease, the more this will benefit future generations of coeliacs.

Defining coeliac disease

Coeliac disease (also known as non-tropical sprue, gluten-sensitive enteropathy, idiopathic steatorrhoea, primary malabsorptive disease and, in the United States, celiac sprue) is a condition in which a person's body reacts to the protein fraction called gliadin, which is found in gluten.

Coeliac disease is an autoimmune disease. A healthy immune system will recognize foods like gluten as being harmless and tolerate them. An unhealthy immune system will not do this and, instead, attack it like it was an infection, causing damage to the lining of the small intestine. This may sound like there is an allergy to gluten, but coeliac disease is not an allergy. While some people can grow out of an allergy, coeliac disease is a permanent condition – it lasts for life.

When a coeliac eats food containing gluten, the lining of the small intestine becomes damaged, so much so that the villi and microvilli (tiny projections on the lining of the small intestine that aid the proper absorption of nutrients) are destroyed to varying degrees, resulting in malnutrition. Figure 1 shows what normal villi look like when proper absorption is taking place. Figure 2 shows damaged villi, which are typical of malabsorption and coeliac disease. As you can see, the difference between normal and damaged villi is often dramatic when viewed under a microscope. In coeliacs, the villi are partially or totally absent and the microvilli are severely flattened or reduced. Enzymes located on the brush border of the small intestine are also drastically reduced. This is a totally different picture to that of a healthy person's small intestine, in which the villi and microvilli are in abundance and resemble finger-like projections.

Removing gluten from the diet results in prompt improvement for all coeliacs, so it is essential to adhere strictly to a gluten-free diet after a positive diagnosis has been made. The small intestine will not heal until gluten has been completely removed from the diet. Once removed, a coeliac's small intestine usually does return to normal, but this can vary depending on how long the coeliac went untreated and how strictly the coeliac sticks to a gluten-free diet.

What causes coeliac disease?

For coeliac disease to occur, the following three factors must be present:

• a genetic potential to develop the disorder

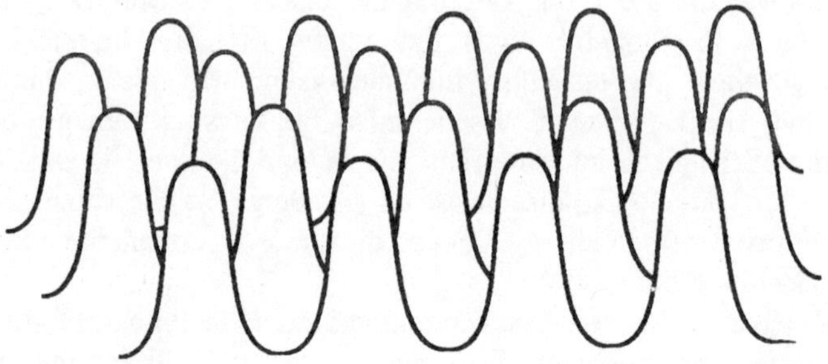

Figure 1 Normal villi.

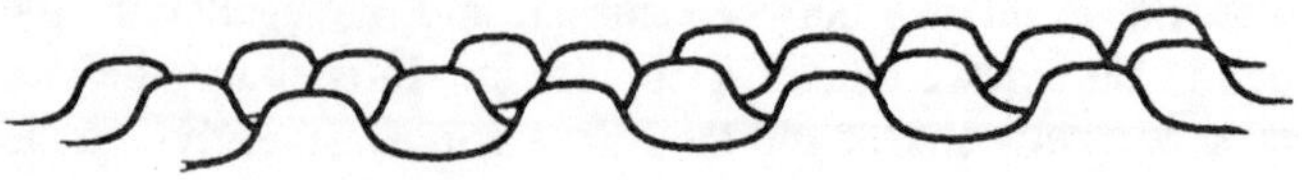

Figure 2 Damaged villi.

- a source of gluten in your diet
- a trigger factor.

If there is anyone in your family who has coeliac disease or a disorder related to coeliac disease affecting the immune system (see Chapter 3 for more details), you will have the genetic potential to develop coeliac disease. What this means is that you have genetic markers, called *HLA subfactors*, which make it possible for you to develop coeliac disease. It does not mean that you will definitely develop coeliac disease just because you have these – other factors must be present for this to occur.

One of these factors is that you must be eating a diet that includes gluten. This is not difficult in today's world of fast food and snacks; many foods people eat have gluten in them. Just think about your daily eating routine and try to count the number of items you eat every day that have gluten in them – bread, sandwiches, gravy.

Even with gluten in your diet, you will also need a trigger factor in order to develop coeliac disease. The following is a list of common trigger factors that have been reported by coeliacs and their doctors.

- A dramatic increase in gluten in the diet. For example, suddenly changing to a low-fat diet, which often means increasing your intake of wheat-based products.
- Surgery, particularly in the gastrointestinal area (such as, the gallbladder).
- After the birth of a baby, when a woman's immune system is adjusting to the changes that occur after delivery.
- Having a viral infection that you don't recover from.
- Psychological stress.

If you have experienced any of theese factors, when they occurred may have been when you developed coeliac disease.

What are gluten and gliadin?

Gluten is a cohesive, elastic protein that is left behind after starch is washed away from wheat flour dough. It acts as a rubbery binder, which is useful in cooking. For example, without gluten, the results of baking would be just crumbs.

Gluten is made up of a mixture of individual proteins. The two main groups of proteins in gluten are called the *prolamines* and the *glutelins*. The most troublesome protein in gluten for coeliacs is the prolamine *gliadin*. Gliadin is what damages the lining of the small intestine. How gliadin harms coeliacs is still not known for sure, but several theories are being considered in Europe and the United States.

As a coeliac, the most important thing you need to be concerned about is knowing which products contain gluten and, therefore gliadin. This is crucial, because gluten can hide in many products. In Chapter 5, you will find out how to be a gluten sleuth.

The genetic connection

If you have coeliac disease, you may be worried about any children you may have also developing the disease. Most studies indicate that approximately 10 per cent of a coeliac's immediate relatives may inherit the genetic markers for coeliac disease. Remember, this means that they have the potential to develop the disease, given a trigger and a diet that contains gluten. It also means that they may never develop the disease. If you find that someone in your family is showing symptoms of the disease and you have been diagnosed as having it, it would be wise to suggest they go for tests to check this out.

Those of Northern European ancestry seem to be more prone to developing coeliac disease than other groups, although it can occur in other races, including North African, Arab and Slavic people. In Ireland, approximately 1 person in 300 has coeliac disease. In the United States, the figure is much lower, approximately 1 person in every 2,500. Europeans are leading much of the research into coeliac disease, and for good reason as it is much more common in Europe than anywhere else.

The disease affects both sexes and can begin at any age, although it affects women slightly more than men. In general, though, coeliac disease is not a widespread disease.

What happens if coeliac disease goes untreated?

If you know you have coeliac disease, be wise and stick to the treatment – a gluten-free diet. Untreated coeliacs can experience a range of medical problems, some of which can be fatal. If you don't know whether or not you have the disease, then you will be one of the many untreated coeliacs who usually go from doctor to doctor searching for a diagnosis. This is particularly common in older people, where the likelihood of misdiagnosis is high.

A great amount of research into the effects of untreated coeliac disease is being undertaken, so ideas are changing, but, in general, untreated coeliac disease has been linked with the following:

- a higher probability than normal of developing malignancies like lymphoma, duodenal cancer and esophageal cancer
- neurological complications, like numbness or even polio-like symptoms
- bone diseases, such as osteomalacia (a softening of the bones) and osteoporosis (a porous condition of the bones usually related to ageing)
- intestinal ulcerations
- refractory sprue (when your symptoms do not clear up on a gluten-free diet because the intestinal lining is beyond repair).

If you are a coeliac who occasionally cheats on your gluten-free diet, you should also consider yourself to be an untreated coeliac. You must not cheat. If you do, the damage to your small intestine continues. All of the medical problems listed above result from this ongoing damage to your system.

Your immune system will be able to put out a finite amount of energy to fight the invader, gluten. After the immune system's energy ceases, it will break down and other medical problems will develop. That is why there is a higher probability that people who are diagnosed as having coeliac disease in their 50s and 60s have already developed other serious health problems than if they were diagnosed earlier. The longer a coeliac continues to eat gluten, the longer the gliadin will eat at them.

3

The connections between coeliac disease
and other conditions

As coeliac disease is an autoimmune disease, it follows that there are other autoimmune system diseases associated with it. These conditions do not develop because of gluten or coeliac disease itself, but, rather, because coeliacs are part of a group genetically predisposed to autoimmune diseases.

Some research suggests that when a coeliac has an autoimmune disorder in addition to coeliac disease, this condition may be a secondary problem, coeliac disease being the underlying condition that permitted the autoimmune disorder to develop. If this theory is true, many interesting questions arise. Would a gluten-free diet help improve a coeliac's other autoimmune disorder? If a coeliac has relatives who have an autoimmune disorder, are they possibly undiagnosed coeliacs whose health would greatly improve on a gluten-free diet? While these questions have not yet been answered by medical science, we must treat any connection between coeliac disease and any other condition seriously.

Skin diseases

The relationship between skin diseases and coeliac disease has received considerable attention. There is substantial evidence that with adult coeliacs, itching *eczema* of various types can occur. Scleroderma has also been mentioned as a disease related to damage of the small intestine.

One particular type of skin disease that has received a lot of investigation in connection with coeliac disease is *dermatitis herpetiformis (DH)*, an intensely itchy skin eruption distinguished by the formation of small red bumps and blisters. These lesions tend to occur in groups, similar to herpes, hence the term 'herpetiformis', meaning 'like herpes'. Most people cannot avoid scratching the lesions because of the intensely itchy, burning and stinging feeling accompanying them. The lesions can be distributed almost anywhere on the body, but they are rarely found on the face, facial hairline or in the mouth. The disease can persist indefinitely and is a lifelong condition.

Some doctors believe that all DH sufferers also have coeliac disease, while others believe that most, but not all, do. What is clear is that most people who have DH have very similar small intestinal linings and immunological findings to those of coeliacs. Also, gluten has been found to have a close relationship with the skin rash that occurs in dermatitis herpetiformis, so when gluten is removed from the diet, DH sufferers show vast improvement.

Conventional treatment for DH sufferers requires that the person take the drug dapsone every day. The symptoms will often disappear within 48–72 hours, but once the dapsone is stopped, symptoms recur. Most people who have DH can avoid taking dapsone when they follow a gluten-free diet. Unfortunately, many DH sufferers, as they often do not experience the severe gastrointestinal symptoms some coeliacs do, feel that going on a gluten-free diet is too difficult, so they take the drug dapsone. The potential adverse affects of being on medication for long periods of time cannot be stressed enough. Therefore, if there is any other less invasive alternative treatment, it should be considered. It is thus highly recommended that all DH sufferers follow a gluten-free diet. In only a small percentage of cases does someone who has DH not recover fully on a gluten-free diet and have to continue taking dapsone.

Multiple sclerosis

Some studies show that there is a connection between coeliac disease and multiple sclerosis (MS) in certain cases. It is not clear whether this is solely genetic or chemical in nature. While there is still much we don't understand about this relationship, some facts are worth considering. Multiple sclerosis is a disease of the nervous system wherein the myelin sheaths (the fatty substance which surrounds nerve fibres like insulation) are dissolved, thus hampering the transmission of nerve impulses. Symptoms include numbness, weakness, paralysis, tingling and burning sensations, loss of balance, poor co-ordination and impaired double vision. The range of symptoms that each individual experiences depends on which specific nerves are involved, so MS is difficult to diagnose, as there is no typical case.

People who have MS have a metabolic defect which prevents them from being able to utilize saturated fats in a normal way. This is similar to the fat malabsorption problem experienced by coeliacs. If this exists in those who have MS, then the possibility that a gluten-free diet may be effective in the treatment of MS must be taken seriously.

There are cases that support this reasoning. Roger McDougall, a well-known British playwright, was admitted to the National Hospital for Nervous Diseases, London, in 1953 and diagnosed as having multiple sclerosis. He slowly became an invalid and for ten years he was practically paralysed and in a wheelchair, hardly able to speak. When he found out a gluten-free and refined carbohydrate-free diet might help him, he tried it, with astounding results. From 1965 onwards, he was able to lead a normal life for someone his age, writing plays again and being physically active. All because he changed his diet? That's what he says.

While there are not always such dramatic results for MS sufferers who go on a gluten-free diet, many do find that the disease progresses more slowly than before. Others find that some, but not all, of their symptoms go away. As MS sufferers' conditions develop over many years, it cannot be expected that their symptoms will just disappear overnight. Progress occurs but it is slow, even on a gluten-free diet, so determination and perseverance are important.

There has been no official endorsement of a gluten-free diet for MS sufferers yet. Unofficially, though, the benefits of a gluten-free diet for MS sufferers cannot be discounted and it's certainly worth a try.

Schizophrenia

There is growing evidence that coeliac disease and schizophrenia appear in the same person or possibly in the same family more often than they would by chance. Children with coeliac disease more often than by chance become adult schizophrenics; and adult coeliacs develop psychoses more often than by chance, too. This does not mean that if you have coeliac disease you will develop a mental illness, but if you have coeliac disease and several family members have mental illnesses, they should check whether or not they also have coeliac disease.

Medical literature on the adverse effects of grain on mental status is controversial and still very vague. In some studies, schizophrenia has been associated with gluten intolerance. While it is unlikely that schizophrenia is a single disease with a single cause, food allergies may play a role in treating schizophrenics. Professor F. C. Dolan has consistently advocated this idea for over 20 years. In 1966, he stated that, '. . . considerable evidence indicates that the major cause of schizophrenia is the inborn inability to process certain digestion products of some food proteins, especially cereal grain glutens. . .'.

There is no way to estimate the magnitude of the relationship between coeliac disease and schizophrenia, but it is important to remember that there is a connection when either you or members of your family suffer from mental disorders.

Lactose intolerance

It is not uncommon for coeliacs to be lactose intolerant. *Lactose* is the sugar in dairy products. Before it can be absorbed, it must be broken down by an enzyme, *lactase*. This enzyme is made at the tip of the villi which line the small intestine. When the lining of the small intestine is destroyed, as we have seen it is in coeliac disease, the body isn't usually able to produce the enzyme to make lactase. Without enough lactase, lactose from dairy products is not absorbed normally, producing acid and gas. The end result is watery, acidic diarrhoea, bloating and excessive gas.

Lactose intolerance should go away when a coeliac follows a gluten-free diet because once the gut heals, lactase will start to be produced again. This can usually take up to six months after you have started a gluten-free diet. If you are lactose intolerant, avoid lactose for the first six months and then ease back into consuming foods that contain it.

Diabetes

There is a high incidence of diabetes in coeliacs and their relatives and so the link between these two diseases is being explored more and more. The American Diabetes Association has even begun to look into this relationship, initiating a study with its diabetic members to determine the prevalence of coeliac disease among them. It is thought that possibly immune mechanisms may hold the key to why diabetes and coeliac disease are commonly linked.

Other conditions

Numerous other conditions have also been connected with coeliac disease. While the stream of new results from research is always changing or refining our knowledge of the disease, there does seem to be a link between coeliac disease and quite a few others.

Other autoimmune disorders – like Grave's disease, Addison's disease, chronic active hepatitis, myasthenia gravis, systemic lupus erythematosus, Sjogren's disease and possibly rheumatoid arthritis – have some sort of link with coeliac disease.

Some research suggests that candida (a systemic yeast infection) and coeliac disease are connected. While coeliac disease is not the underlying cause of candida, according to some theories it can contribute to the development of systemic yeast. Dr Lloyd Rosenvold, in his book *Can a Gluten-free Diet Help? How?*, says that

> The putrefactive processes in the bowels incidental to the maldigestion and malabsorption present as a result of the coeliac disease, furnishes in the intestinal contents an ideal culture medium for the propagation of the candida yeast organisms. A perfect, warm, moist and putrefactive environment – ideal for the rapid multiplication of the yeasts.

The connection between coeliac disease and autism (a mental condition that starts in childhood and makes them turn away from the outside world and other people) is also being taken seriously by quite a few people. A far greater number of autistics than could be explained by chance have coeliac disease or food intolerances. Also, abnormal responses in autistic children to gliadin have been reported, which has lead to support groups being formed, even over the Internet (see Appendix I).

Keeping up to date with new developments

Every day, research is going on and we continually learn more about coeliac disease. You can keep up to date about new research by reading the wealth of newsletters and magazines available through coeliac societies, associations and groups throughout the world or by jumping on the Internet. The information is out there when you start looking.

4

Talking about coeliac disease

The stories in this chapter provide examples of how coeliacs are coping with their condition and how their family member's cope. As everyone copes differently, you may not see yourself in every story, but it is still valuable to share other people's unique perspectives on what it's like to have coeliac disease. There is a lot of power in people's experience – it can enlighten us with thoughts we never thought of, make us laugh at common experiences and teach us to appreciate the ups and downs of living with a lifelong disease.

'How am I going to live without bread?'

Rachel, 29, had recurring anaemia from the time she was small. The only typical coeliac symptoms she had experienced before diagnosis were severe fatigue and occasional stomach pains. Eventually, after a bad bout of anaemia, she was referred to hospital. A haematologist checking her sample of blood was the first person to suggest she may have coeliac disease.

I had one endoscopy and then I was put on a trial gluten-free diet. I had to go back for another endoscopy three months later to see how I was repairing. They decided there and then that it was coeliac disease. Although I'd been sticking strictly to the diet, I hadn't really recovered properly, but the doctors told me I had to stick to the diet and eventually it would repair itself. They kept suggesting more endoscopies, but I didn't find it very comfortable so I didn't go back for more. Also, when I went back for the second endoscopy – after I had stuck to the diet and been so good – and they said it really hasn't done anything, that shattered me as well. I thought, I've been so good for three months and they couldn't even praise me for that and I thought, I tried so hard. I wanted to go out and binge on bread. I really did, I wanted to just say, 'sod you!' and have a loaf of bread.

When I was told to go on the gluten-free diet, at first I was devastated and I felt very angry that I couldn't have what I wanted to have. My whole life I was surrounded by bread. Big chunks of bread. Bread and butter. Anything like that. It wasn't so much cakes and biscuits and pastries, but it was the bread, that was the first thing that crossed my mind, 'How am I going to live without bread?' I lived on it. I was very depressed and I wasn't a very nice person to know at that stage. At work I went through a bad patch for about a month coming to terms with it.

It was very difficult to explain my feelings to my husband at the time. When I started on the diet we'd have separate meals. My husband would have meals I could have, but, of course, because he doesn't have to, he didn't want to do that all the time. You know, he's missing his foods as well. He can have them, and that's fair enough. At first I found it difficult to prepare things for him that I couldn't eat, but now it's old hat. My husband was just glad to have somebody to talk to again as, before the diet, I would always come home and go to sleep and I was grumpy and tired. On the diet, he saw I was changing and becoming more alert. I was changing into a different person, so he was quite happy about knowing what I had.

One day I just turned to myself and said, 'I'm going to have this for the rest of my life. It's either like it or lump it'. So it was just a matter of, get on with it. It could have been worse. My brother died eight years ago and I thought about that. At least I can control my health with a diet, which isn't that difficult. Other people have diabetes and have to change their diet and they cope.

My parents were very supportive of me on the diet. Though sometimes my Mum used to vex me because she would call every day and say, 'What did you have today? Check the contents'. It was non-stop. She'd get me lots of gluten-free things and they'd invite me for meals with them and would make sure there were lots of things I could eat. To start with, she wouldn't let anyone else in the family have anything I could have, which actually annoyed me. Or she wouldn't serve cakes or biscuits or bread because I was there. Finally, I told her just because I can't have them doesn't mean to say nobody else can have them.

I have adjusted to people eating things in front of me that I can't eat, but it still hurts now, seeing a lovely fresh loaf of bread in front of me and there's my father or husband or brother tucking in and I think, 'Can I have one?' They just laugh now, they know that I'm just joking. But I'd do anything for a sandwich. I know a cheese and pickle sandwich sounds so boring, but to me that is just my dream. Fresh slices of bread and a bit of cheese and pickle between them!

A couple of my friends felt sorry for me when I was diagnosed, but I think that's because of the way I was acting. Because I was so cross and depressed about it they felt sorry for me because it must be difficult. But my friends and family have all rallied round and so they've helped me through it.

I don't tend to go for many of the gluten-free substitutes. I find they're a waste of time. Everything has a powdery, malted-milk biscuit aftertaste, so I'd rather go without. I do get the bread on prescription and the chocolate chip cookies aren't bad. Even making a dish and substituting the gluten-free version didn't feel right to me. Knowing I was having a certain dish and the gluten-free version didn't taste the same seemed to make the diet worse for me.

I did feel well after I went on the diet. My dad asked me if I felt well and I said, well, I don't know what well ever felt like. I knew I felt very different. I had more life in me. I wasn't going to bed at 6 or 7 in the evening and sleeping through until 7 in the morning. I could stay awake, which was a big thing with me. I'm not sure how much feeling better was also relief of actually having a diagnosis as well as the diet working. If I hadn't been diagnosed and I had a baby, I don't know how I would have coped because I would have been sleeping more than the baby. The diet has definitely changed me.

I have an eight-week old baby now. I had no problems at all during my pregnancy, except I craved bread throughout! I was on iron throughout the pregnancy, but there were not really any special precautions because I am a coeliac.

Getting gluten-free food in hospital when I had my baby was a bit of a rigmarole. They knew that's what I needed, but the usual sheet came round for what you want the next day and I ticked a salad, but they had salads like pork pie salad or something that I couldn't have. So I asked if I could have a salad just with cheese and they said 'Oh yes, of course!' But it took them until I was leaving to sort it out. I kept telling them I can't have this because I'm gluten free and they said, 'Oh yes, you are, we know that', but the food that came round wasn't gluten-free. My Mum brought me gluten-free biscuits. Other than that, I didn't eat much. There were a few things on the menu I could have, but not much. I had the same thing every day. But it was just a few days and I knew I could have what I wanted when I got home. And I had a little baby, so food was the last thing on my mind!

Cutting out bread from my diet was very hard. I was brought up on bread, and with every meal. We'd have bread to mop up the gravy, so to just stop automatically was difficult, but I think it's probably good that I don't eat so much bread any more.

I put weight on with the gluten-free diet because what I was eating I was actually absorbing. Before I was diagnosed I could eat anything and not gain weight. Then, right after I went on the diet, I soon put a stone on, but now I don't gain weight.

I have a lot of energy now. I just want to go out all the time, walking. I want to go out and be doing something – I don't want to be sitting around doing nothing, which was how I used to be as a teenager.

Lunchtimes at work were the hardest when I first went on the diet. I used to always take sandwiches with me, but when I went on the diet I couldn't think of what I could eat. I was having to go to the canteen at work and I found all I'd eat was salads because that's all I knew I could eat. If I went out for the day on the weekend, that was also difficult, especially finding a snack to eat. There isn't really a snack I can have except maybe a jacket potato, which to me just gets boring. The few snacks I can have, I get bored with. Most quick snacks have bread or something in them that's not gluten-free. That's the biggest problem I've found. And there's only a limited amount of time I have in the day to prepare any food and I don't want to prepare snacks. So I've sort of come to a standstill with it. I grin and bear it now and do without most of the time.

Going out in the evening was not a problem because I could always safely eat steak and chips or meat and vegetables and salads. That's what I tend to stick to. Now that I'm working nearer home, I can come home and have *my* bread, toasted, or a small salad. There's only a limited amount of things I can have quickly – and you get into that, 'Oh, I had that yesterday. What else can I have?!'

If I go over to someone's house for a meal, I tell them I can eat a salad or meat and vegetables – anything that hasn't been processed in any way. All my family and friends now know, so I'm always the exception, as it were. Desserts are very difficult. Usually people serve a pastry or something like that – but I can only have ice-cream or jelly. I feel like I've gone back to my childhood, eating jelly and ice-cream! But it's more difficult on other people – I've never been a big dessert eater anyway. The hosts always find it difficult, they think I'm not eating enough. They always want to give me more of something. I don't know what it is, but they all say, 'Are you sure. That's all you want?' But, well, that's what I usually have.

I hated in the beginning feeling the centre of attention. As I said, my Mum used to prevent anyone else from eating anything I couldn't eat while I was around. The same goes for special occasions and family get togethers. Everyone asks, 'Well, what can you have?' And I say, 'Well I'll just pick out what I can have and don't worry about me. I'll just get on with it.' Now many of my friends know about my condition and there's no problem, but initially I felt awkward. At lunchtime I just felt like going home and doing something for myself. I didn't feel like I wanted to join in because I was always the odd one out. If there was a big spread, with lots of food on the table I'd have a big plate of things that I could have put on the side for me so that I'd have something. People would save me bits of this and that of foods I could have, and that was very awkward.

What helped a lot was communicating with my family and friends and saying, 'Look, I'm not that different, just let me get on with it. You don't watch anybody else and what they're eating'. So, it then became a mutual agreement to let me get on with things and it's a lot easier now.

I haven't been on any long holidays yet, just a few days away in the UK on a self-catering holiday. But I think if we went abroad, I used to eat salad stuff anyway – I never used to eat that much – so I don't think it would be too difficult. And if I did have something that I wasn't suppose to have, then it can't be helped. If I wasn't sure what was in it and there was nothing left on offer – well, I'd have to eat, wouldn't I?

I have cheated. I tend to get headaches and feel lousy and sluggish the next day or two, but I don't do it too often and, when I do have something, I know that I'm not going to feel a hundred per cent the next day. One thing I miss is pizzas and my husband likes his pizzas, so I might have a little bit of his pizza – just a mouthful or two, just to know what I'm missing! But I don't go out and buy things purposefully. If my husband has something and it smells or looks so good, I've got to have a bit and he says, 'Well, if you're not going to feel well it's up to you', but sometimes I have a bite. I don't go out and eat a whole portion of anything. I don't really regret cheating. I live for the cheats!

My husband came home yesterday and he just wanted something quick to eat and he said, 'You've eaten all the cereals!' and I said – Oh, I have?! I buy them for myself because I can't have toast in the morning! And for a snack he just has a piece of toast. That makes me angry, that there's a small variety of things that I can have so when there's none of it around he complains, when there's all those things he can eat, so he should not have my things to eat because he can eat anything. That gets me cross.

Since being on this diet, I have really noticed what ingredients are in different foods. I never had any idea what was in foods, I just bought whatever I wanted to eat, completely ignorant of what was in it. But because I really have to watch all the labels now, it really has brought to light what I can and can't have. I never knew what I was putting into my body, whereas now I do and I think I'm a lot more healthy. Now I'd rather go for something that's fresh instead of something that was processed.

I wouldn't say anything has changed because of eating a gluten-free diet. I've got back into a routine. Because I know what I can and can't eat, things don't affect me that much now. But to start with everything revolved around food for me. I had to be careful about what I ate and was learning about what I could and couldn't eat. The book from The Coeliac Society that tells you what you can and cannot have and all the brand names, that used to be like my bible. It went everywhere with me. But now I tend to have things I do myself rather than buying processed products. It's changed me for the better, really.

I wanted to feel like everyone else. I hated feeling different. It took a few months before I started to feel OK about it, but now I feel great.

'If you stick your head in the sand, nobody's going to take any notice'

By profession, Maureen is a state registered nurse. Her husband and father are doctors as well. So, as she puts it, 'You would think my coeliac condition would have come to the fore before I was 49!' As a child, she always had a huge, bloated stomach. This continued into her adult years. Then, at 48 years old, she began to have chronic diarrhoea, was losing weight, couldn't eat and felt dreadful. As her doctor was on holiday and she felt the covering doctor was of little help, she sought private medical help. After lots of tests, they found nothing. Maureen now felt as though she was withering away. The only other option presented to her was to use a gastric camera. Reluctantly, she agreed and, to the surprise of even the doctor, it was found that she had coeliac disease.

Now, because I am starved of gluten, if I have so much as a grain of gluten, the reaction is major. My stomach goes like a board and starts to hurt and I cannot go to the toilet. My body seems to tie up in a knot. Then I don't eat for at least two days. I go on fluids only or maybe a bit of food if I can stomach it, but normally I don't feel like having anything at all. It takes about 24 – 48 hours for my gut to release the spasm and then I'm all right. And I usually tell the person who has given me gluten in no uncertain terms what they have done to me. Usually it's hotels.

For my work, I go to lunches that are held at hotels. Some hotels are good and understand what a coeliac can and cannot eat, but the last time I went to a hotel that I normally trust, they served me what they said was leek in cream, but it was not leek in cream, it was leek in cream sauce. And two hours later I knew it had gluten in it, so I went back to tell them the next day and I gave them a list of the foods that I can eat from The Coeliac Society and I said, 'Be very careful because the next coeliac you poison could be a child'. They are usually horrified. They have no idea and don't understand gluten-free. They just think you're being fussy and you're possibly a difficult client. But when I explain in no uncertain terms what exactly happens to me, they then change their mind and hopefully they're more careful. With very susceptible coeliacs you only need to use the same bread knife from ordinary bread into something that a coeliac eats and it's contaminated and away you go.

When I was told to go on a gluten-free diet I can remember saying to my doctor, does that mean I can't drink? I drink wine, and my brain couldn't quite tune in at that point, but of course it's lagers and beers that I can't have which doesn't worry me in the slightest. I used to occasionally enjoy a lager when it got hot, but then when I look back on it, as soon as I would drink the lager, up would come my stomach. So I don't know why on earth it took 40-odd years to be diagnosed.

My husband's family is confused about this diet. They don't know what to do with me. It doesn't really worry me in the slightest, but I do tell them, 'For goodness sake, don't put any flour in anything that you're going to give me'. Or I take my own food. I don't mean to be insulting, but I'd rather take my own food and know that I'm safe eating it than end up with a bellyache and hours of diarrhoea.

Socially, we don't go out in the evening very much so I haven't hit the problem of going out to people's houses. If we go out to lunch with friends, I've usually spoken to them beforehand and then it's usually the dreaded salad. I will look like a rabbit soon. Because people don't really understand exactly what gluten-free means, it's easier to tell people to just give me a salad and I'll be fine. And for God sake don't put any mayonnaise on it until I look at the bottle!

Having to check food labels in shops has been a nightmare. I've had a long-standing relationship with a major supermarket chain near my house. Because I shop there all the time, I got to know what I can eat. We used to sometimes have made meals from the supermarkets, but, of course, that had to stop straight away because they put modified starch in everything and you don't know which starch it is.

About six months after I was diagnosed, I was shopping on a Saturday morning and I saw the Manager walk past as I was looking at two bottles of pasta sauce and I said, 'Right young man, come over here and explain to me why you can't put on your bottles which starch is in this product'. And he said, 'Why?' And so I sat there and explained to him for an hour and a half – poor man! After this hour and a half conversation, he was completely blown away, he had no idea of the coeliac condition, he had no idea what difficulties I was having. Although this supermarket does publish a coeliac list, I'm sure they don't really realize exactly the problems coeliacs have and how many there are. He then said would I like to come and meet one of the marketing people when they come down next month? So I did, and I brought with me the Chairlady of the local Coeliac Society. We sat down and they offered us coffee and said, 'Would you like a biscuit?' And I just looked at him and he said, 'You can't eat that can you?' And I said, 'No, I can't'. He said, 'Oh, what can you eat?' And I said, 'A banana'. Then he said, 'What about those rice biscuits?' and I said, 'You eat them and see what they're like'. So he went and got a packet off the shelf and said, 'They're dreadful!' And I said, 'Yes, they are. I don't want them, thank you. Please, just get me a banana!' So, he and this marketing chap walked around the supermarket with us and I tore things off the shelf and said, 'Look! modified starch! That's not helpful, so I can't eat that because I don't know what starch it is. Why don't you put on it which starch it is? Is it rice starch, wheat starch, corn starch, potato starch – which one?!' And he said he had no idea what kind of starch it was and I said, 'Well, it's about time you sharpened your ideas up, isn't it?' There must be lots of people out there who are diagnosed coeliacs, not registered with The

Coeliac Society, who spend all their time looking at labels like me or know there's no point in buying anything from the supermarkets because they don't know what's in it. I told this Manager that their supermarket sales would go up a hundred fold if they labelled things properly. Also, if they thought about it, but obviously they haven't and it's about time they did, why don't they do made meals, clearly labelling which starch is in them, and then the Trust hospitals and maybe even some of the private hospitals might want to purchase the meals for coeliacs when they're in hospital? A lot of hospitals don't have diet kitchens any more. He hadn't thought of that. We then moved on from that and apparently when their new labelling comes out they are going to clearly label all the ingredients in detail on every product. Hopefully, when the new labelling comes out, all the ingredients should be clearly marked. So that's one step forward.

I use a breadmaker and a gluten-free mix and I have fantastic bread. The breadmaker is totally and utterly automatic. I love it. Of course, while it is very nice, it's not like bread with gluten, but I tried all the other commercial gluten-free breads one can buy and I thought they were pretty bad. It was just a sort of batter with muck. You'd put it in the oven and it would come out like glue. I'd sit there and think, 'I've got to eat this for the rest of my life? I can't be doing this, I've got to find another way'. But I can imagine that there are people out there who haven't got my assertive manner who may be very depressed about being a coeliac and eating gluten-free.

When I go to my local supermarket now, I'm known by name and they see me with my bag of carrots and gluten-free stuff, and the number of checkout ladies who now say, 'I'm a coeliac and thank you for doing what you're doing. It's amazing'. They haven't bothered to join The Coeliac Society and they just live on fruit and vegetables and meat and can't be bothered to say anything because probably their lives are too full or they just feel they have to put up with the lack of available coeliac items. This is crazy because if you stick your head in the sand nobody's going to take any notice and they'll just go on their happy little way and think, 'I'm all right, I can eat all these foods' and tough luck for the coeliacs. Well, that's not the case because there are so many thousands of coeliacs out there either undiagnosed or who haven't registered with anybody, so nobody knows exactly how many there are. If there's a huge public awareness, then I think big supermarkets' sales will go soaring because people will know they can buy products there that they haven't been able to eat for years because they've been terrified of the content.

The people I initially saw when I was diagnosed were helpful, but they just gave me a few lists of things that I could and could not eat. That was it then. There you are, now go away and live on this revolting diet of gluten-free crackers and fruit and vegetables and that's it. And come back in six months and have a blood test and thank you very much and goodbye. That's what I was told. Having always enjoyed my food, I thought, 'poo poo' now I can't have this, that and the other and that's not going to be very good for me – I shan't be a very happy person.

I'm a survivor. I've just had so many things happen to me over the years I wasn't going to let this diet depress me. It's just one of life's little hiccups. A lot of people have said to me, that it must be terrible not being able to eat gluten. And I say, 'Well, I'd rather have the little c than the big C'. That I can cope with, I don't think I could cope with cancer.

I make people laugh when they say, 'What can you eat?' when they see me standing there eating a Mars bar. And I tell them, I'm not a great sweet eater, but I can eat a Mars bar. I can eat the big Mars bars and I can eat the snack size Mars bars, but I can't eat the fun-size Mars bars because the first two are made in this country, but the fun-size Mars bars are made in Holland and they've got wheat in them. There's a bit of what seems like useless information, but it's crucial for coeliacs to know this. Things are not clearly marked, you have to look. If you are used to eating Mars bars, obviously the easiest thing would be to have a fun-size bar because they're one bite or two bites. Luckily I never had a fun size bar, but I would have obviously soon known if it had gluten in it because I would have reacted. I would have assumed Mars bars are made the same throughout the country. Coeliacs need to know this.

Being on a gluten-free diet has affected me the most when we eat out. For example, my husband and I went out to one of our local restaurants last night. They are fine. They understand totally that I can't have anything with gluten in it and they make the sauces for me with cornflour and make sure I don't have any flavourings that contain wheat. So I know I can go to this restaurant and I know I'm looked after and there's no problem. They know for dessert I can't have cake or a biscuit, so they brought me extra fruit and they don't make a fuss. In other restaurants I say, 'I can't eat that, please get me something else' and they look at me as if I had just grown another head, but it doesn't bother me because I'm me. But I'm sure there are people out there who don't go out to eat because they're afraid they might have a reaction and you're made to feel like you're something odd. I can speak to anybody and don't feel intimidated. If you're an introverted sort of a person, it must be much more difficult, but that would never apply to me. I always take the opportunity at a restaurant to inform them exactly what coeliacs are, so that when they meet another one they don't regard them as something different.

Years and years ago if anybody had cancer it just wasn't talked about. Now it is talked about. Some coeliacs do talk about it, but a lot of people don't because they are frightened of the reactions. A lot of coeliacs have told me that they can't be bothered mentioning they're a coeliac. And I say, 'Why?! Why are you frightened of saying, "No I can't eat that"? Why be frightened because you can't help it. You're not being difficult or fussy. It's just that the food makes you ill!' You don't say to a diabetic, 'Have this lump of jam' do you? So why should coeliacs be treated any differently. Diabetics can't help it, and coeliacs can't help it. They don't go out of their way to be downright difficult!

I think, if anything, I get a bit frustrated in my day-to-day life. For instance, I fly into a petrol station to fill up the car and all I see is sandwiches and God knows what. Years ago I used to grab a sandwich and that was fine. Now I think, 'Damn, why haven't they got any fruit?!' If I know I'm going to be out all day, I'll usually take one of my little sandwiches on gluten-free bread with a Mars bar and some fruit and cheese. Sometimes, if I'm out longer than I anticipated, I'm caught without food and there's no one who sells any fruit!

I used healthfood stores the first weekend that I knew I was a coeliac. I went down to the local healthfood store and bought some ready made gluten-free bread, which I think is the worst bread I've eaten in my entire life. It was vacuum-packed. It was hideous. I didn't find the person in the shop very helpful, but I live in a place where I doubt there are many coeliacs or people who would say they were coeliacs. She just pointed to the gluten-free products. But I don't go to healthfood stores very much because I don't need to. I buy ordinary food and adjust it to what I can eat. We tend to eat a lot more home-made things than we did before.

My daughter's very funny. She'll pick something up when we're shopping and say, 'Can we have this Mummy?' and I'll say, 'Yes, you can' and she'll say, 'Oh, you can't have it. Never mind!' It's sweet. She understands the problem I have and is quite helpful. If we're out for the weekend she knows there's a pot in the freezer box that's mine and she knows it's not a question of not wanting to share it – I can't have anything else! The other weekend, when a couple of friends came over, my pot of food was on the top of the freezer box and somebody said, 'May I have a bit out of that pot?' and my daughter said, 'No you may not. You can have some out of this other pot, but that is my Mum's, don't eat hers!'

You have to bring your own pots of stuff all the time. If you're out all day, sometimes a little van comes around selling hot sausages, fish, chips. But it's all in bread and if I wanted some chips I don't know if they will have been cooked in oil or in something that contained bread, so I can't be sure of that. If I don't take my own food I'd end up very hungry by the end of the day. I don't feel awkward at all opening up my own pot of food.

When I was diagnosed last year, after three months I went back to see the doctor who diagnosed me and he asked me how I felt and I said, 'I feel fine' and he said, 'No you're not, you won't feel fine for at least a year. You don't know what it is to feel fine'. And now it's virtually a year later and I agree with what he said, I had no idea what it felt like to feel fine.

I'm nothing like as tired as I used to be. I'm 50, but I frighten 20 or 30-year-olds. I work full time, I sell private medical health insurance, I help look after my daughter's pony, I have a horse lorry, so I drive her everywhere with that, I load the pony, I'm flying up and down with the ramp – I don't regard myself as the normal 50-year-old because I don't feel my age now.

'It scares me that I'll have to be on this diet for the rest of my life'

At 17, Phil is a coeliac trying to cope with all the pressures of staying gluten-free and leading an active social life with his friends. He was diagnosed with severe anaemia when he was eight – so severe, in fact, that one doctor in hospital commented that he had never known a Western child to be so severely anaemic. For several years, Phil took iron supplements and had regular blood tests to check his iron level. All this time he was very skinny. Then, around the age of 13, he began to suffer from chronic headaches. This led to

34

another series of tests and, eventually, after much confusion, he was diagnosed as having coeliac disease.

I didn't really know what a gluten-free diet was all about, I just knew I wasn't supposed to eat anything like bread and cake – the things that you eat every day. I didn't think it was fatal if I didn't keep strictly to the diet, so I wasn't too upset. I didn't think it was going to be for the rest of my life. Then the dietitian told me I could never go off the diet. I didn't say a lot, I just sat there and thought, 'That's it'.

It's hard when you just want to go for a bite to eat because everyone else can have a pizza, but I can't and there's not much else on the menu I can actually eat. Sometimes I just eat pizza because there's nothing else, but if I can wait I'll either not bother or have something like chips. When I go out with my friends and all that's available for me to eat is chips, it's hard. My friends all know that I have to eat gluten-free and they're all all right about it. If I eat something I'm not supposed to, they'll often stop me, but it's hard.

My family was very supportive. I had one last meal with gluten after I was told to go on the diet and then that was it – my family has only made gluten-free meals for me at home since. I didn't feel very different at home, I had basically the same meal as them. They eat pizza and I eat it, too, but with my gluten-free pizza base.

I started feeling better on the gluten-free diet after a couple of weeks – the headaches went away. Now, when I eat gluten again, I get a headache a day or so later.

It scares me that I have to be on this diet for the rest of my life. I think, 'I'll be able to do it, but it's going to be hard'.

'At first I suppose we all watched him while he was eating, like we were paranoid he'd eat the wrong thing'

As the mother of a teenage coeliac, Phil's Mum, Sally, also had to cope with Phil being a coeliac.

The first time they diagnosed him with coeliac disease I felt relief because by then I was beginning to think that something more life-threatening was going on. It was a relief to be told it was a dietary problem. Then I thought, 'Oh no, this diet will change my whole way I do shopping'. I couldn't just go in and pick up any old thing any more. At first it was an absolute nightmare because it literally took us ages to go around a supermarket because you had to look at everything. Now there are a lot more products about with gluten-free marked on them, but it's still very, very limited. One thing I find intensely irritating, we religiously buy the brands we are told are gluten-free, but the next time we get the list, they're taken out. There we were, buying all this stuff, being so careful and then in the next booklet it tells you not to buy what you've been buying! I know it's frustrating for everyone.

I got the booklet from The Coeliac Society of all the foods you can and can't eat and what brands you can eat because that was the other nightmare, you would look up baked beans and think you could eat baked beans, but you could only eat certain brands of baked beans. It became a hassle because I always shopped in one supermarket, but when I went to buy hotdogs the brand that Phil can eat is sold at a different supermarket, so I would pop over to the other part of town. So not only do you have a limited number of things you can eat, but it is also limited by brand name.

After he went on the diet, I did tend to feel guilty for eating anything because he would say, 'Well, it's all right for you, you can just go to the cupboard and eat anything'. I felt like it laid a guilt trip on me. I tended to wait until he was out of the house until I had a biscuit. I tried to get stuff that he could eat as well, but there comes a point where you can't just buy him a cake or a packet of biscuits, so I felt guilty about helping myself to a biscuit. If he saw anyone in the family eating anything with gluten, he'd say, 'Well it's all right for you, you rotten lot!' Not meaning it in a nasty way, but I did think it must be awful not being able to just get a biscuit out of the cupboard if you felt a bit peckish.

At first I thought there's absolutely nothing I make that he could eat! I didn't realize my cooking had so much gluten in it and it stunned me what he couldn't eat. It seemed like it was virtually everything to me, even down to the gravy that I do. He couldn't have it. I was thinking, well, never mind, I'll just cook him a proper meal every day like potatoes and vegetables and things like that and then stick a bit of gravy on it. Then I realized, hang on, he can't have that so I had to thicken every gravy with cornflour. He tends to do that himself now while I'm doing everyone else's gravy, but at Christmas and holiday time things can become a problem. His friend's mother took them for a

Christmas lunch and he rang me up from the place they went to and told me what he had to eat, realizing that he couldn't have the stuffing which was the obvious thing and I asked him if he had gravy on it and he said 'Yes' and then it dawned on him that he shouldn't have had it. So, in effect, that wiped out all the other things he'd avoided. I thought maybe one mistake wouldn't be really bad, but the doctor said he only needs a tiny, tiny little bit of gluten and it could undo everything.

At the moment I worry that Phil doesn't take it seriously enough in terms of the long-term effects because at 17 when you're talking about middle 30s it seems like a lifetime away. And at 17 you think you're immortal, nothing is going to touch you. Although he understands that he shouldn't be eating it and 99 per cent of the time he's brilliant – and I don't know if I could do it – I know for a fact that within this last month he hasn't been that good, particularly when he's out. I know he does drink beer a little and he's not allowed any form of beer. I've tried to tell him that the doctor said there is only so many times that your bowel will repair itself and there's going to come a point in your life when it possibly won't. I don't know if from that point his bowel is repairable, not repairable, if he's going to have to wear a coloscopy bag or if he going to die – I honestly don't know, but I have said to Phil it could be potentially fatal and he could be in big trouble. And I know he understands, but I think, 'Well, he's only 17 and I'm talking about what seems a whole lifetime away'. I know he's normally very good in sticking to the diet, but it's the fact that it doesn't take much to undo it.

I've said to him to take food with him to work because he can't keep eating chips. The only other thing he can sometimes get at work is a baked potato with cheese. I want him to take some gluten-free rolls with him, but have you ever smelt these rolls? They're not nice.

I've used the flour and done sponge cakes for him so when we have a cake he has one. We made pancakes with his flour and he said they were brilliant. Now every time I get home he's cooking pancakes! It was at least something different that he really, really liked and it was as near to normal as possible.

I think the holiday time is one of the most difficult times for him because he can't eat Christmas cake, Christmas pudding. His friend's mum was really good and went and bought the kinds of foods Phil can eat for when he goes around there, but most people don't even think about the little things they serve to eat, like gravy. Someone will tell me what they're making and I say that's all right and then they go and coat it with gravy. Then the meal's ruined for him.

The family reacted very well to Phil's new diet. At first I suppose we all watched him while he was eating, like we were paranoid he'd eat the wrong thing. He'd pick something up and we'd all go 'No!' And he'd go on for five minutes asking if he could have just this one of this or that. Now I don't think the family ever even thinks about it. His brother will sometimes tell me if Phil hasn't been eating the right thing, but, apart from that, everyone has just accepted that that's the way Phil eats. Nobody avoids eating a cake any more, even if he's sitting there. If I know somebody's got a cake, then I make sure he has got something in its place. It might not be as nice as a cream cake. I generally tend to avoid puddings unless they're ones Phil can eat as well. I just don't intentionally buy it. I don't like to have any food with gluten around that are easy snacks because there have been times when he comes home late and he has gone to the cupboard and there are no biscuits he can eat or something quick and then I know he'll have a couple of the biscuits he shouldn't have.

I do get scared about Phil's future. I know all his friends know that Phil has coeliac disease and on the whole they're quite good, but he doesn't like being around people who don't know him very well because it's uncomfortable for him to say he has coeliac disease. He started work and he hasn't told anyone there. He can get something cooked for him, but at the moment he hasn't told anybody so he tends to have salad or chips all the time. Sometimes I think he has accepted he has coeliac disease, but when it comes to actually saying he is a coeliac to other people and he can't, I wonder if maybe I'm just assuming he has accepted it when he actually hasn't. I don't think *I* would have a problem with anybody else knowing, but I'm not 17. It wasn't until I said something about him eating something he shouldn't eat that he then eventually told his girlfriend he's a coeliac. But I know he told her in a way that put the diet down, like it didn't matter if he didn't stick to it rigidly.

'I was there as a ready-made dustbin to eat anything she decided she shouldn't eat'

James was the husband of Kathleen Ogborn, to whom this book is dedicated. As the spouse of a coeliac, he explains Kathleen's condition and how they both coped with her gluten-free diet. Kathleen eventually developed cancer of the transverse bowel and it invaded her stomach. She died, peacefully, at home in 1996.

Kathleen originally started to feel ill in the late 1970s, when we lived in Nigeria. That illness was diagnosed as thyroxine deficiency. The specialists dealing with her thyroxine deficiency were completely baffled that she wasn't getting better, so she eventually – after a lot of tests and changing the dosage of her thyroxine many times – was sent to see a gastroenterologist. From the time we came back from Nigeria, she had chronic diarrhoea and then it got worse. That was the main symptom she had. She was also anaemic all of her adult life. On two occasions she had to go into hospital suddenly with anaemia, sickness and pain and they just couldn't find anything specifically wrong with her that would cause the symptoms she had.

She was diagnosed in 1990, at the age of 66, with coeliac disease. Her reaction was not to bother about it, live with it. Either she would or I would make a loaf of gluten-free bread. She wasn't going to be preoccupied by her diet and she kept herself very busy with other activities and preferred to do that than to worry about having a nice-tasting diet. She was absolutely meticulous about having a gluten-free diet because that's what worked.

It took about three months for her to recover her normal health and strength. She was noticeably better. When we were out, there were things she could eat that were inherently gluten-free, but she had to be very careful when going out to a restaurant to avoid things that had been basted with flour. But once she was better she found that, in terms of her physical health, she could eat the occasional dose of gluten without any disastrous effect. The main effect of having gluten was that her diarrhoea temporarily became violent. That was the main embarrassment of her disease. She continued to have some diarrhoea even after the gluten-free diet, but it was much better.

We went to Uganda after she was diagnosed with coeliac disease. We usually found that we could get a gluten-free meal on the airline and, by being sensible, she could avoid sauces. Of course, she soon found out if she'd made a mistake and eaten gluten. One meal she ordered on the plane was free of everything. It was incredibly uninteresting – it had nothing in it except energy I suspect, which didn't really matter. The other thing Kathleen often ate – simply because she liked it and knew a bit about what was in it – were Asian meals. They taste nice and often are gluten-free. In Uganda, we ate sorghum and millet-based meals. She didn't find it very difficult to cope going away, partly because, if necessary and she was stuck with no food to eat, she just starved. I was there as a ready-made dustbin to eat anything she decided she shouldn't eat. I could eat anything that she couldn't. The only thing the diet did to me was to enlarge my already too expansive figure. Kathleen was a very sensible girl and she coped.

Because at home we had lots of vegetables from the allotment, both of us were very happy to make egg-based things. We ate lots of vegetables because we ate them from our garden. It's terribly difficult if you're not eating a home-grown fresh diet because you tend to get gluten in everything ready-made. One of the sad things she found is that she had to take very little alcohol because it made her feel bad.

If you are not able to cope, it's because *you* are not able to cope. Coeliac disease was not really a problem she couldn't cope with.

'You have to do what you need to do to get well and not think that much about it'

Cathy, 39, was always poorly as a child and didn't grow well compared to the rest of her family. She comes from a family with four diabetics. She had various sicknesses throughout her life and whenever she got something, it was always worse than normal. Around the age of 34, she began to have chronic diarrhoea, suffered this for two years and was eventually roughly diagnosed as having irritable bowel syndrome. Then, one night, she couldn't breathe and was admitted to hospital with pneumonia and severe anaemia. She wasn't getting better and no one knew what else could be wrong. After she kept refusing the sandwiches they were giving her in hospital, one doctor asked, 'Could you be allergic to bread?' Almost immediately she was given an endoscopy and it was confirmed that she had coeliac disease.

My first reaction to being told I had coeliac disease was relief that it wasn't something very serious and it could be controlled with a diet. Then there was this sort of horror about what I could actually eat! Luckily, there was a nurse on duty at the hospital who had coeliac disease herself, so they sent for her and that was quite useful. She talked to me about it and gave me the name of The Coeliac Society person in this part of the region and they were most helpful because all the hospital gave me was a sheet of paper that said, stay off this and that and I was thinking, 'Well, what can I actually eat?' There didn't seem to be a lot left.

As I never liked bread, that wasn't very difficult. As a child, my friends used to say to my Mum, 'Oh, your daughter's not eating her sandwiches!' I just didn't like them. I suppose sometimes you know instinctively that some things make you sick.

I felt better within a few weeks of going on the gluten-free diet. I didn't feel tired any more, I was a lot brighter, my skin got better, I put on weight and even have to watch my weight now. Suddenly I've got curves! I have a different attitude on life. My stomach problems have gone away completely, but I have to be very, very careful – I can't even breathe it in! I've had four incidences where I've come into contact with gluten. The first one, my husband gave me some mackerel in a tin and it wasn't the one I should have eaten and just from one mouthful the whole week I had diarrhoea and was sick. I just have to sit on the toilet with a bucket. I can't do anything else. My body just gets rid of it as fast as it can, I can't even walk straight.

The next time I got sick was when we went to a new restaurant while on holiday. We had a long chat with them and I said I didn't want anything with a sauce and we explained I was a coeliac, so it came down to that I could only eat the fish. Well, it was only later that evening that we realized the fish must have been slightly coated with flour and then grilled. So I was very ill and unfortunately I spent the whole holiday in bed or on the toilet with a bucket. I'm not sure if this is related, but at that same time my eyesight went peculiar. The doctor said he has never known this to happen before, but now I have one pupil larger than the other.

The third incident was at a crêpe shop that I'd been to before. They do buckwheat crêpes and I went there with a friend, told them I was a coeliac and they said the buckwheat pancakes were 100 per cent gluten-free. We ate them and I was fine. Then I went back with my children two weeks later and I just ordered a meal with buckwheat pancakes again. When I left to pay, I said to the owner it's so nice to be able to go out to eat and not worry about what's in a meal and he just looked at me in horror and said, 'Oh no, you're the woman who is gluten-free!' And I said, 'Yes, why?' And he said, 'Because the gluten actually sticks things together well, when you make buckwheat pancakes they will stick together better with gluten'. He said that as he knew last time that I was coming in, he hadn't made the mix with gluten, but usually they do. I didn't have a violent reaction to them, but I did get sick. And I also came out in a red, itchy rash all over, which I hadn't had before. It lasted about a week.

The fourth time was making playdough at school where I teach little children and I got sick from breathing it in. I didn't think that would cause it, but it did. I wear a surgical mask now when I do cookery at school with the children. The children think it's hilarious, but they know I'm allergic to it so they accept it.

My family and friends were just glad they found out what was wrong with me. In the beginning, at home we had to get rid of a lot of things and I always walked around with this booklet telling me what I could eat and what to avoid. The whole family eats mostly what I do now. They still have bread, they have their own pasta, their own pizza bases. Everything that is not gluten-free is one colour and my gluten-free stuff gets a different color, so everyone knows what they can eat.

The hardest thing is going out for meals. We don't any more, really. Everywhere you go, the meal you are offered is in a sauce or has a gravy or it's pasta. The salads that are ready-made for lunch all have a pasta base or a sauce, so I just can't have them. You find you're starving yourself to death sometimes! Or if you go to friends' houses, they get so uptight about what they can give you to eat and they go out and buy things that they think are gluten-free or wheat-free, but I still can't eat them. The other day I went to a friend's house and she bought me a rye bread and pumpernickel, which I couldn't eat. It's embarrassing. I tell them before I go not to do anything special and then they still do it and I still can't eat it. That same friend bought a ham, but unfortunately the ham was breadcrumbed around the outside. Of course, she never even thought of that. So I like to say don't bother and I'll bring the food I can eat with me, which is what I normally do. I bring my own gluten-free bread and then tell them to get me any plain meat. I keep saying plain food, hoping that they do, but occasionally they don't.

When I'm in a restaurant they think you're picky. I was in a restaurant the other day and I told them I wanted a steak, but make it with nothing on it. They said, 'No problem', and it arrived with cauliflower and a cheese sauce on the side. I said I couldn't eat it and they said they'd take it back and scrape the cheese off, but I had to say, 'I need a completely clean plate and clean piece of meat'. And she said, 'Why?' And I said, 'Because I'm allergic to wheat'. 'What if I just scrape it off?', she asked again. And in the end I have to make it sort of really seem bad and tell them I'd be in hospital if I eat it, just to get the message across that I will actually be ill. Some people say, I don't like it, but could eat it. With coeliac disease a lot of people are going to be very ill if they do eat it. So many times in restaurants I'll explain everything and I get a polite, 'Yes', but then when the ice-cream comes along I get a wheat wafer stuck in it. You have to overemphasize everything and, in the end, you wonder if it's worth the bother. You end up not eating at the restaurant table while everyone else is eating.

Most of my friends know I'm a coeliac and are very considerate. I have a friend who always has a plate of gluten-free biscuits just for me, so it's quite nice that they do it. I've got used to people doing these things for me and because I feel so much better I can joke about it that I've got a diet that's actually making me healthy. You just accept it.

Our holidays are often now self-catering. We did go away to a place that wasn't self catering and every day I'd go to the head waiter at breakfast and ask for their evening menu and I could choose what I was going to eat. If there wasn't anything there, then they would make something up for me. It was nice, but I still didn't trust them. Unfortunately, you just can't always trust people to follow your instructions to the letter. Every single meal tends to have something in a sauce, so I usually end up eating green salad and fresh fruit. It gets a bit annoying when you're paying £20 for the meal and that's all you can eat of it! The restaurants often are prepared to make it separate for me, but I really don't want to put them to the trouble because they have enough to cope with. Plus, sometimes you talk to one person and another person makes it, so that person hasn't heard your whole explanation of what you can and cannot eat. I know I can get food I can eat, it's just the thought of having to explain it. We went to a Chinese restaurant and I asked them if the food had any flour in it and they thought I was talking about *flowers* as in roses. They finally got the message, but sometimes it takes so long it doesn't seem worth the hassle. I can normally eat chips when I go out, if they're not cooked in oil with batter, so they're safe. When I get meat at the supermarket, I have to ask that they wash the cutting board down before they cut my meat because they may have cut other breaded meats on that board and then the little bits of bread can get on my meat. They're very good if I explain things, it's just I don't always want to put them to the bother.

I can't eat anything at lunchtime because I work in a school and they just have school dinners, which I definitely can't eat. I take my own food, like gluten-free breads and pastas. Initially it was difficult because people would say, 'Why are you eating this?' Or the children would offer you crisps at breaktime and you feel a bit guilty about saying, 'No thank you'. You feel as if you're embarrassing them by refusing something you're offered. And quite often the children will make me cakes at home with their mums and I come in and see a cake sitting on my desk and think, 'Oh! Great!' At the end of term, they give me boxes of chocolates and they often want you to open them right then and start eating them. I offer them all round and hope that they come back to me with none left! I do explain to some parents, but it's not easy to say no. I'll often say I'm going to put it in my bag to eat later.

Everything that we eat now is fresh, never from a tin. It wasn't really such a big change for my family because we did eat so much fresh food already, it's just making sure that any processed foods we do use are the right products.

I don't cheat at all. I was too sick. I did always have a sweet tooth, so I do miss cream cakes. When the children go to the cake counter and pick out a nice piece of cake and then the person behind the counter says, 'Anything else?' I have to take a deep breath before I respond. I've never been able to make a decent cake with the gluten-free flours I use. I keep changing the flour, but it's not the same, so I don't eat cake at all now. I experiment with gluten-free recipes once in a while, but not often. I may buy a breadmaker because I'm eating a lot of bread now and I heard they're quite nice and easy. I also miss my Guinness! I didn't drink a lot, but I liked drinking. Wine will do, I guess.

I'm healthier, fitter and happier now. I don't really get sick any more. My husband was always taking days off every month to take care of the kids because I was too sick. Now it's once in a blue moon that he has to take off work. If you don't feel well all the time you do begin to feel a bit depressed, but now I know I'm just like normal people with my health, I can do just about anything I like. I got my strength and my weight. I was almost like a walking skeleton for many years, so now I'm incredibly stronger. And I had a second endoscopy about a year after the first one and it was completely normal. I think if you feel healthy your whole life takes on a different attitude. You don't shout at the kids as much. Now I love having children around, it's all fine. You have to do what you need to do to get well and not think that much more about it.

'Very occasionally I say to myself, "I'm going for it today"'

When Carol started her nursing training, she thought she had irritable bowel syndrome. That was about 30 years ago. Now, at the age of 56, Carol looks back and realizes her health problems go back a long way. At that time, her bowel troubles were just intermittent – never really incapacitating where she had to stop work, just inconvenient. After she had her children, her bowel problems seemed to improve and were less noticeable because she was home-based. Then, in her mid 40s, after changing her diet to more wholegrains because she quit smoking and thought she might gain weight, she began to feel unwell. For two years, her appetite got smaller and smaller, her diarrhoea persisted and she enjoyed her food less and less. Eventually she went to her doctor and demanded she have comprehensive blood tests. After noticing her folic acid level was extremely low, her doctor immediately had her tested for coeliac disease and it was confirmed. There are eight diabetics in her immediate family.

At that point, when I was diagnosed, I was greatly relieved because I assumed I must have got a tumour of the liver. I am a nurse and I've seen this before and thought it is bound to be a liver cancer with these symptoms. The thought of doing anything about it was too horrendous for words and I thought I'd rather not know.

The doctor who diagnosed me said he could start me off with folic acid and calcium and iron and I'd feel a lot better for that, but he said I'd feel even better, and it's better for me, to go on a gluten-free diet, but he'd have to personally say that he could not give up his bread or biscuits so, if I'd like, he would keep me going on supplements. He said the choice was mine. So, I started off with the supplements and felt a great deal better – I could walk up stairs easily again and lead a normal life again, but I still didn't go on the diet, which is difficult because you have family and relatives that you're sometimes cooking for. About six weeks after being diagnosed, my husband went away for work for six weeks and there was no one else in the home so I thought, 'That's it, I'm going to go on a gluten-free diet and see what difference it makes to me'. And I've never turned back. Within the first week I felt a difference. One of the most disturbing feelings that I had before I started the diet was it felt as though my stomach was full of mercury. It felt heavy, it felt bloated and as I walked it seemed to move about heavily. It was a horrid feeling. Within a week that had gone and my appetite had improved and I was eating more sensible foods. Initially I just cut out bread, but gradually I cut out other cereals. I went onto potatoes and rice and vegetables and meat and fruit. Bit by bit, I'd introduced other gluten-free things that I could eat and, by the time my husband came back, I had got my own gluten-free bread and crackers.

I miss the cakes and pastries that I used to make. I grieved over bread for quite a long time. I almost felt angry at other people who were eating it. Not now, I've just forgotten about what it tastes like. Occasionally a good loaf of bread will make me feel down. My husband and I now go our separate ways with bread and every now and again I say he's absolutely revolting and disgusting because there's a wonderful bread shop that does overnight bread, it's slow-rising, old-fashioned bread that smells wonderful and the rest of the family eats it and I can smell it a half a mile away! I can smell wheat now, if we have it in the house, I can smell it.

I haven't been very tempted to eat gluten, but very occasionally I'll say to myself, 'I'm going for it today'. About twice a year, something will tempt me and I'll say, 'That's worth a week of diarrhoea for'. I've cheated once in a while – partly as a test just to make sure I'm not on this diet for nothing – but within two days the diarrhoea starts.

After I started this diet, I had to be very careful that I didn't get constipated, for the first time in my life. And I put on weight, as I'm enjoying my food a lot – different food, of course. I found some very good gluten-free crackers, so I can still have my magnificent Brie and Stilton cheese in large quantities.

I'm a bit of a cook and I like natural ingredients – I don't like processed things – so it wasn't as bad to go on a gluten-free diet for me as it could be for some people. If I actually went to Marks and Spencer and bought their precooked meals all the time and heated them up it might be a big problem, but I've never been tempted in that direction. I rather enjoy cooking from basics, so then the gluten-free wasn't that bad. Going out for meals I have to watch a bit, but we either do Chinese or Indian, which are fairly safe. Chinese and Indian tend to use either corn or lentils for thickening, and if we go to a very expensive restaurant, I send a word down to the chef and ask if a dish has gluten in it and they're very good and helpful. Obviously if you go into a cheap restaurant, they're going to say it doesn't have gluten when they may not know. In fact, I got caught in error in a pub the other day. I was having a jacket potato with coleslaw in it and I said this coleslaw is very odd, the mayonnaise base is different – it's very nice and I'm enjoying it. And 36 hours later I was on the toilet. The mayonnaise wasn't gluten-free. Some brands are and some aren't and you have to be careful. There are now a few that I know and I stick to.

Cooking a meal when all my children are around hasn't been a problem at all. I make something with potatoes. It is hard to make a good white sauce now because cornflour doesn't work as well as wheat flour. So I tend not to do those kinds of sauces. I just alter my recipes a bit and it works.

I do travel. Overseas it gets slightly dodgy, but I do work my way around situations. We went to Florence last year and got to the hotel to find that their buffet breakfast was actually rolls and jam, but eventually I found that they had yogurt and they did have a cereal if I wanted it and they had cheese. I took packets of my gluten-free bread so if I got stuck I could always have the bread with butter for breakfast. But, on the whole, we try to go to hotels where they do an English-type breakfast because, although I don't normally have a cooked breakfast, I'd go for ham and a scrambled egg instead of bread and marmalade. The coeliac bread is pretty disgusting, but toasted they're just about acceptable, so I sometimes have that. Overseas, the language problems can get quite funny, but we get there.

My friends were horrified when I went on a gluten-free diet. They don't like feeding me any more – they are frightened of it and cannot get their heads around it. Not all of them, but many. They would turn to me and say, 'Well you do eat cheese, don't you?' There was just this total incomprehension as to what gluten was in. It actually shook me that people were so unaware of the contents of food. People get terrified that they'll give you the wrong thing. I find there are fewer people who think about my needs and it has cut down the number of people we will drop in and go round for a meal at their house. You know, if I'm at someone's home at lunchtime they would be saying, 'Stay and have a spot of lunch', and now they're saying, 'I wonder if I've got anything you could eat if you stayed for lunch?' It makes me feel dreadful, pinickity. I feel like I'm making a fuss. I don't feel any more comfortable now than when I was first diagnosed with coeliac disease. On an ordinary everyday level, with my family, they understand that I'm totally not a fussy person, they know that. My kids managed very well. They were out of the home already. Now they come home and Mum's no longer making pastries and biscuits. It's different.

Always requesting special food in different situations is difficult. I would rather pick my way carefully through a menu than make a fuss about it. There are times on holiday when I find a few things to eat, but if we were staying in that hotel for a week, I wouldn't want to eat that same food for a week, so I will then start asking questions and making it known that I'm a coeliac. If every restaurant you go into you have to say, 'I'm a special case', I just try to find something simple, even if it means eating a steak, which is not something I'd normally order out to eat because it's so easy to make at home. On a very limited menu, I find it's the easiest thing to order without making a fuss.

I always have a banana in my bag and, if needs be, I eat a banana. At work I don't normally have lunch, but there are some times when there's a catered conference where there will be just a pile of sandwiches. That's when I pull out my banana. In those situations I don't feel very uncomfortable because we're all medical people and they know me and we're like family. Elsewhere, people will look at me and say, 'Oh, you must be slimming'. And I laugh because oddly enough I'm actually putting on weight!

If people are interested, I'm quite happy to talk about it. I'd really rather people talked about it than just said, 'There's another oddball'. My Mother is the worst about that. She really believes that I'm just being stupid and no daughter of hers could have this strange disease and I'm just being picky. She'll always ask me, 'Are you going to have some of your funny flour, some of your funny bread?' It's pretty awful. She has now become diabetic and I feel like saying, do you want some of your funny sugar? To her, diabetics are sick people, coeliacs are stupid. My sister who's a diabetic is a 'poor sick thing', while I should just 'get on' and stop being so picky. I don't feel like I want to go around being thought of as sick, and I don't feel sick.

'With having candida as well it was very difficult'

Ruth's physical health began to deteriorate rapidly after her second pregnancy. She was on antibiotics continuously for two years, trying to get rid of various problems that plagued her health. She had chronic diarrhoea and was told by her doctor she had irritable bowel syndrome. When her bowel didn't improve, she was sent on a ten-week social phobia course. Eventually, at the age of 31, she went to see a clinical ecologist, skilled in identifying allergies, and he suggested she undergo tests to see if she had coeliac disease. After it was confirmed that she had coeliac disease, she still wasn't greatly improving on the gluten-free diet. Eventually, she was also diagnosed as having candida. There are seven coeliacs in her immediate family.

I don't cheat at all. If I have something with gluten in, it's because it's an error. Sometimes, even in my own kitchen, I found that I reacted to gluten going into my skin. If I'm doing pizza bases for the rest of the family and I have to knead dough, I wear gloves now because I do find that it will go through my skin and I get very tired and out of breath. And I know a lot of coeliacs are the same. I only found this out last year when I went to my consultant and he said he thinks I am highly susceptible to any kind of gluten in any form, so it might be a good idea to wear gloves if I'm cooking. Once a week I would do a batch of pizza bases for the kids and my health didn't feel right, so I kept thinking, 'What on earth is wrong with me?' What I do now is I get the kids to make the pizza bases, which is fine. Usually when I feel bad I can trace it to some form of gluten. Cooking with flour and breathing it in sometimes will also make me feel bad.

The food list that The Coeliac Society produces is brilliant, but I had an incident the year before last where I was eating crisps – a certain brand of crisps that was on their food list – and then I found out about six months later that it had been taken off the food list. But I get afraid that things like those crisps I was eating may have had gluten for the previous six months before it was picked up by The Coeliac Society and taken off. It's very difficult. So I tend to stick to fresh foods because of that.

Within a year after starting the gluten-free diet I felt better, but with having candida as well it was very difficult because half the time I didn't know if what I was feeling were coeliac problems or candida problems.

Support is a crucial part of how I got better. For me what's

49

important is being able to say, 'I feel like this and do other people feel like this?' That's all anybody with any disease is really trying to find out. It's nice to hear people with the same disease talk about their symptoms – you stop panicking so much.

If I relapse I get diarrhoea, pain, passing out. Really full-blown. I would go to bed with hot water bottles and that's just from some little bit of gluten getting into something I ate. I now know they can transport crisps on floured conveyor belts. Something you wouldn't dream of. I couldn't believe the things I'd been eating and then discovered, 'Oh, now that has gluten in it!' But you get used to it. I don't have the need to cheat at all because of how bad I get. So that stops me. I have never cheated and probably never will. Some people I know who have coeliac disease were diagnosed quite quickly and it sometimes makes me want to cry. I think, why did it take so many years to diagnose me, and for me to get so ill, and yet this person, they got a little bit of diarrhoea and didn't feel quite right, go to the doctor and soon after find out they have coeliac disease?

If I get down and feel off a bit, then I go and read some book on health or the *Crossed Grain* magazine from The Coeliac Society. It gives me something to read and then think, 'Well, I'm going to be OK'. It gets me through the bad times.

I still cannot manage eating fruit – I react with bowel problems, headaches, my legs get achy, so I stay away from it. Plus, to check on what food intolerances I may have, a friend of mine who has candida does muscle testing on me and I do it on her. A clinical ecologist taught us how to do it and we both find it very accurate. The clinical ecologist saved my life. I would not have been able to identify all of my food allergies on my own.

The gluten-free products are OK. It's the same thing with anything, you brainwash yourself into thinking that it tastes like a 'normal' food product would do, so they're OK. It's like the first time I had soya milk it really made me want to vomit. Now to me it tastes like milk. So you become brainwashed!

I have my prescription bread, toasted, and I make sandwiches. I have my goats' cheese. Put in some lettuce and away I go. That's my sandwich. But it's not like getting my teeth into a crusty bit of French bread that has just come out of the oven and smells really gorgeous. I'll never be able to taste that again. Also, because I can't have milk, there is only one gluten-free bread that I've found that doesn't have milk in it. That's a bit of a pain as well. I tend not to have the gluten-free biscuits because they are just packed with sugar and even my husband has had them and said they taste like pure sugar – it's just too sickly. But I make my own biscuits with rice flour and dates because I can make them to my own requirements and it's much healthier because it's not all that sugar. I take my biscuits everywhere – just in case I'm somewhere and there is nothing for me to eat, I always know I have a couple of biscuits in my bag. If I don't keep something in my bag to eat, I tend to regret it.

Every party we go to you can guarantee it will be all pastry or bread-based, so I've got no chance of eating. We went to a party the other week and the only thing I could have on the table was melon. Even the salad dishes had bits of croûtons and things like that. Unless I go to my Mum's, and she's very good – she'll keep a salad on the side for me and she'll make sure there's stuff on the table for me – but most people don't have the first inkling. I'll say, 'I can't eat something because it has pastry in it' and they'll say things like, 'Well, have a slice of gâteau!' I usually just laugh now and think, 'Oh yeah, they're trying to kill me off!' People don't understand what gluten-free means. It's surprising how many people don't realize that flour is in a biscuit! When you say you can't eat flour, they tell you to have a biscuit. And when you say to them, 'Do you think a biscuit would be cooked with flour?', they say, 'Oh, possibly'. People have no idea, they're so ignorant. I was so surprised.

My friend takes the comedy side and will say to me, 'Do you want one of these?' even if it has flour in it because she can't remember what I can and can't eat. It's quite funny how different people react. Some just panic completely and think, 'Oh my God, she's not eating anything. She's not going to be happy. She's not enjoying herself because she's not eating'. And then I feel a bit frustrated because, before I go to any party, I make sure I have had a proper meal so I'm not going to be in a situation where I am starving hungry.

Some people just keep going on and on and then it feels like they're making an issue that you're something different. I'd rather people ignore the fact that I'm eating something different. It's all right once in a while, but when you go to someone's place and they go on and on about your diet and all these people are just looking at you I think, 'Oh my God, just swallow me up, do we have to go through this again?' I tend to tell people I don't know that, 'I don't eat such and such because I don't like it', and people will accept that, but if you tell them you're a coealic, then there's all this mumbling and then you've got to have a big discussion about it and a debate and open it up for questions and I get very tired of it because I've gone past that. I just want to get on with my life now and enjoy myself, I don't want to have to explain to anybody.

'I've known no other diet except a gluten-free one'

Stephen grew up with coeliac disease. He was poorly as a child – his stomach was constantly bloated and he was always sick. By the age of three, he was diagnosed as having coeliac disease and put on a gluten-free diet. He immediately began to thrive and, up until now, at the age of 38, he has had no major health problems.

I've not known any other diet except a gluten-free one. As I was growing up, I just decided I'm always going to be on a gluten-free diet. At school sometimes it was difficult, like for things like pancake day, I couldn't eat the pancakes, so I was given a Milky Bar to eat. For school dinners, my friends could have fish and chips and I used to have boiled fish. I found that very difficult to cope with at that time, but I didn't cheat at all going through school. As I grew up, I didn't find being gluten-free a problem and I was able to discuss it with my friends. If we went out for a meal, it was all right for me to say, 'I'm allergic to flour'. That was the best way for me to explain it to people, that I could never have anything with flour in it, and they really didn't see it as a problem.

At 23 years old, my new doctor asked me if I ever thought about trying to come off of the diet. I said 'No' because people have told me that I'm going to be on it for life and that was OK with me. He proposed that I try to eat a slice of toast every morning, ordinary toast, and I didn't want to do it. The fear of making myself ill was too great, so I never tried it. I do sometimes have a meal now and I don't worry about what I eat and I don't seem to suffer. I've gone out and had fish and chips with batter on the fish and there doesn't seem to be a reaction. Even so, whenever possible, I will still never touch gluten, but if I go out for a meal I won't say any longer that I'm on a gluten-free diet, I'll have things with sauces. I do like all the sauces on the foods. Now when I'm out with friends I don't make a big deal about it because I do appear to get away with it whereas other people I speak to are very sensitive, so it does make me wonder if I can go completely off the diet.

I still won't touch ordinary bread because I have my gluten-free bread that I'm used to. My friends at work will sometimes have a bacon sandwich at lunchbreak, but I couldn't do that because I've always had my own bread and couldn't face eating ordinary bread. If I'm eating a meal with a bit of gluten in it that's not like looking at a slice of bread – I'm conditioned not to eat bread.

At work, we had a canteen and I went to see the dinner ladies and told them I'm on a gluten-free diet and they knew exactly what I was talking about and they always used to tell me everything in the meals and sometimes they would put me on a special meal. It was great. Now the canteen's shut and I have my gluten-free sandwiches.

I only found the diet difficult when I was younger because I was very conscious that I was different, but as my friends were aware of the diet, they were always conscious of what I was eating. They'd always looked after me. As I grew up I had my parents looking over me telling me what I could and could not eat, so I didn't stray from the diet, but when I left home it was more of a challenge.

When I was younger I did sometimes feel like I was missing out when we'd go for a pizza. But then I'd often take my own pizza base and take it down half an hour before we'd go there and they'd put all the topping on it, so it was great, I got my own pizza, which I think was fantastic. I used to feel self-conscious about it, but not at all any more.

I'm just not used to having cakes with my coffee or biscuits, so I just don't miss it because I grew up like that. I personally think you just have to stick to the diet if you're a coeliac. Sometimes my health doesn't feel great and I have to think, 'What have I eaten in the last three or four days?', but, generally, I feel very healthy.

I probably cheated as a teenager once in a while on fast foods. I would never have a hamburger because of the bread. Sometimes after sport there was a buffet and if there was nothing I could eat I would have a sandwich and just eat the filling if I was hungry and then I'd put the plate back with the two slices of bread on it. I don't think my friends really thought about the fact that I was eating anything different, they just knew I won't eat certain foods and wouldn't make a big deal out of it. Even though I'd be hungry sometimes, I wouldn't make a big deal about it.

If I'm going away for the weekend, I will take foods I can eat with me – bars of chocolate, pieces of chicken, eggs – especially if I know it would be a fast food situation, so there's no problem.

Quite often, when I say I'm on this diet people say they know someone else on the diet, whereas years before nobody had ever heard of it. My job has always involved meeting lots of people and they offer me biscuits with my coffee. At first I explained why I didn't want a biscuit every time, but it was going over the same ground every time. In the end, I just said, 'No thanks' and I just had a coffee, so I didn't have to say anything else about it because otherwise I'd have to explain everything about being a coeliac. People were interested, but it's tiring.

When I'm on holiday, it's pretty obvious what I can and cannot eat and I always feel I can usually get a meal that is gluten-free. I do try to stick to meat, potato and vegetables, which are safe. The sauces are the hardest really. My kids usually eat anything that's on my plate that's not gluten-free.

I get the prepacked gluten-free loaves from the chemist, I don't really miss things with gluten and so I just carry on. It's really not a hassle. The only way the diet bothers my wife is that my Mum did more gluten-free cooking than her. The problem with gluten-free products is that if you don't eat it fairly quickly it usually dries up. I generally have to have a fresh loaf of bread every day.

I did taste ordinary bread and it was much nicer than gluten-free. There's no doubt about that. Just the texture is more moist. I didn't feel like I was missing that much. But there's no point to eating ordinary bread.

Turning stories into action

Are you ready to get started on a gluten-free diet? The chapters that follow provide you with strategies to succeed on a gluten-free diet.

5

The importance of a gluten-free diet

Food as your medicine

How lucky you are! You have a condition that can be treated by eating the right foods. You don't have to take a drug for the rest of your life that might cause all sorts of physical side-effects. Eliminating the foods harming your body has no side-effects, except to make you feel better. Food is your medicine. You will heal if you eat the right foods, but eating the wrong foods could cause havoc.

As a coeliac, you will have to eliminate foods containing gluten from your diet. You might also have to eliminate other foods temporarily while your small intestine recovers and cannot absorb other foods properly in the meantime. Taking the power of food seriously is your first step towards better health.

Being told to change your diet to feel better is a foreign concept to most people. For some, it is frightening because it places the responsibility of wellness and healing on them – the doctor cannot make a coeliac better by giving them a pill. If you are a coeliac and you do not stay on a gluten-free diet, you won't get better. It is up to you.

There have been many books written on using food to feel good. In the Western world, unfortunately, most people don't take the phrase, 'You are what you eat' seriously. We eat and eat without considering the effects of the foods entering our bodies. When we have a headache, we take a pill to 'cure' ourselves, continuing to eating the same diet. When we have asthma, we puff on our inhalers, continuing to eat the same diet. When we feel chronically bad with any disease, we look for a quick way to solve our miserable condition. With all the immune-based diseases, which are affecting more and more people, moving towards *conscious eating* – that is, thinking about what foods you're eating and what moods you may be feeling as a result – is crucial if you want to feel good inside and out.

Coeliacs have a unique opportunity to become conscious of what they're eating. It has been scientifically proven that you must avoid foods that contain gluten. In doing so, if you're consciously eating, you will, hopefully, become more enlightened about what you're putting in your mouth every day and your diet will be healthy. The body wants to feel good and stay healthy. Eating good foods is a positive step in this direction.

What is a gluten-free diet?

On a gluten-free diet, coeliacs cannot eat anything that has gluten in it (see Chapter 2 for a definition of gluten). The smallest trace of gluten in something a coeliac eats can damage their small intestine, sometimes to a great extent, so coeliacs must be aware of what ingredients are in the foods they eat. The following lists give you guidelines as to what you can and can't eat on a gluten-free diet. Just reading the lists, though, is not enough; as a conscientious coeliac, you must keep up to date on what is and what is not gluten-free and always *read the labels* of every food item you buy that is not fresh. For guidance on which brands of particular foods are OK, contact The Coeliac Society and obtain a copy of their food list (see Useful addresses at the end of the book).

Foods to avoid on a gluten-free diet

- *Grains, flours and breads* Wheat, barley, rye, oats and, possibly, millet and buckwheat. Be careful of breads and rice cakes that contain millet and rye as ingredients. Also, beware of anything with malt added, as this is usually barley malt.
- *Vegetables* All tinned vegetables should be considered suspect, unless you know for sure they are gluten-free and do not contain preservatives, stabilizers, emulsifiers and a food starch with gluten in it. Any vegetable that has had anything done to it to alter it from its natural state (it has had a sauce poured over it, it has been marinated or fried, for example) should be checked to make sure that what is on it is gluten-free.
- *Fruits* Again, if you're eating fruit that's not fresh (say, tinned), it's best to be sure that the brand you're buying is gluten-free.
- *Meats* Don't eat luncheon meats, prepared sausages, any meat that is breaded and tinned meats containing preservatives.
- *Cheeses* Avoid cheeses that contain preservatives, such as cheese spreads and dips, unless you know the preservative is gluten-free.
- *Drinks and juices* Do not drink any instant coffees, instant tea, instant drinking chocolate or ground coffees that contain grain. Regarding alcohol, avoid all beers, ales and anything made from grain, like whisky, bourbon and most liqueurs. Avoid processed fruit drinks that could have additives in them that contain gluten.
- *Salad dressings* Unless you know the contents and are sure all of them are gluten-free, avoid all commercial salad dressings.

- *Soups* Most tinned soups, soup mixes and gravy, in powder or cube forms, are not gluten-free. Only use those you are sure are gluten-free.
- *Desserts* All products prepared with grains are not allowed, as are ice-creams and cones that contain gluten and all commercial mixes for cakes, biscuits and other desserts.
- *Sweets* All sweets that contain grains are not allowed. You must be sure that they are free from stabilizers that contain gluten as well.
- *Miscellaneous food items* Watch out for some curry powders, dry seasoning mixes, ketchups, mustards and horseradishes, chewing gum, vinegars, margarines, any flavourings made from alcohol, soy sauces made using wheat or MSG and white pepper in restaurants (it is often mixed with white flour to make it go further).

Foods that are allowed on a gluten-free diet

- *Grains, flours and breads* Rice, corn, arrowroot, soya beans.
- *Vegetables* All fresh vegetables. Some tinned or frozen ones.
- *Fruits* All fresh fruits. Some tinned, dried and frozen.
- *Meats* Fresh meat and some tinned.
- *Cheeses* All cheeses, except some brands of processed cheese.
- *Salad dressings* Some commercial brands are gluten-free, but most are not. It's safer to make your own.
- *Drinks and juices* Freshly brewed coffee without added grain. All fruit juices, but beware of fruit drinks which are processed and could have preservatives, stabilizers or emulsifiers added. Most wine, brandies, rum and tequila are gluten-free
- *Soups* Home-made broth with fresh, gluten-free ingredients added.
- *Dessert* Home-made puddings (made using cornflour, tapioca and rice and gelatin) and some ice-creams and pudding mixes.
- *Sweets* Most jellies and jams, sugar, honey and some commercially made sweets, but check before you eat them!
- *Miscellaneous food items* Herbs, salt, spices, nuts, chocolate, most yogurt and eggs.

Becoming your own food expert

In general, if you eat a diet full of fresh foods, you should have few problems going on a gluten-free diet. Initially, you may have to replace some of your usual foods with gluten-free ones, but it won't be very difficult. If you live on a diet of mostly processed foods, however, it will be a greater challenge to switch to a gluten-free diet, but you can do it.

While it would be healthier if everyone ate a diet of fresh foods (and easier for coeliacs), if you want to buy processed foods, you must be absolutely sure that what you are buying is gluten-free. Bear in mind, too, that many manufacturers alter ingredients slightly with each batch they prepare, depending on the ingredients they have available. Also, processed foods are often transported on conveyor belts, which may be sprinkled with flour or contain remnants from the last batch of food on the conveyor belt, that wasn't gluten-free. The Coeliac Society publishes a very useful food list, which is updated every six months. It also has a hotline number members can call, which advises coeliacs about any products that may have to be taken off their food list because the manufacturer has not been able to make a product that is consistently gluten-free. If you buy processed foods, you should check this list often (see Useful addresses for the address of The Coeliac Society).

It is also important to do your own investigating. Read labels. Let me say that again with a bit more emphasis: *read labels*! Every food product should have a list of ingredients on its label. Unfortunately, some labels are vague or inaccurate, like indicating that a product has starch in it but not saying which type of starch it is. Don't let this get you down. Many times, reading the labels can eliminate a lot of the foods you can and cannot eat. It is less wise to rely on supermarket lists of products they say are gluten-free. Some supermarkets produce these lists, often compiled by employees who have limited knowledge of the coeliac diet, and produced at such lengthy intervals that some of the products which were gluten-free at the time the list was compiled are no longer gluten-free. When in doubt about any product, it is best to follow the Coeliac Society's food list as it is compiled by experts on coeliac disease who have the most up-to-date knowledge of which products are gluten-free.

The key is to always *think coeliac* when you go shopping or are out to eat.

What to expect after you start the diet

Most coeliacs begin to feel better on a gluten-free diet within one to three weeks of starting it. Many times coeliacs feel dramatically different, experiencing normal health for the first time in years.

As your small intestine heals and becomes able to absorb all the food entering it, your appetite grows because you're feeling better and the result could be weight gain. For many coeliacs, this will be the first time in their lives they have had to watch their weight. Food may seem to stick to you like never before. If you eat a healthy diet of whole foods, then you should not have serious problems with weight gain. If you eat processed foods, loaded with calories, you will find you can no longer eat and eat and eat without gaining weight. Weight gain occurs because you are overeating, not because you're eating a gluten-free diet. Eat sensibly and you won't gain weight.

Cheating

Don't cheat. It's really not worth it. If you were not too sick before you were diagnosed as having coeliac disease, you may be more tempted to cheat than those who were very ill. It doesn't matter how sick you were before you were diagnosed, however, if you have coeliac disease, the potential to develop more serious diseases if you still eat gluten is something you must consider before you say, 'Oh, it's just this once' and have a slice of wholemeal bread.

An 'on again, off again' attitude to a gluten-free diet is also harmful to your body. Imagine you stop eating gluten for six months, the villi on your intestinal lining begin to regenerate and then you eat gluten 'just this once'. If you are lucky, the lining of your small intestine will be able to recover from this abuse a few times, but, eventually, if this process is repeated too many times, scar tissue will develop on it and these tissues will finally refuse to heal and regenerate. When this happens, your body is in trouble and you may end up with major health complications, of the like mentioned in Chapter 2.

Ensuring you get the nutrition you need

Your nutrition is not at risk if you eat a gluten-free diet. To maintain good health, you need to consume adequate protein, fat, carbohydrate, fibre, water and essential vitamins, minerals and trace elements. All of these can be obtained on a gluten-free diet. Good nutrition depends more on eating a well-balanced diet than on whether or not you're gluten-free. Whole foods are always healthier to eat than processed foods.

The follwing list gives you some suggestions for gluten-free foods that contain protein, fat, carbohydrate and fibre.

- *Protein* Fish, eggs, meat, tofu, pulses.
- *Carbohydrate* Maize, rice, raisins, sultanas, honey, potatoes, bananas, gluten-free pasta.
- *Fat* Butter, gluten-free margarine, cream, nuts, oils.
- *Fibre* Beans, root and leafy vegetables, brown rice, dried raw apricots and figs, fresh fruit.

If you make sure you're eating foods from these four areas, which is not difficult on a gluten-free diet, then your nutrition should not suffer.

When you're not feeling better

If you've been on a gluten-free diet for several weeks and don't feel any better, you need to take the following three steps:

- check your diet again for any hidden gluten
- consider the possibility that this is due to food intolerances
- go to your doctor for further tests.

Checking your diet

Many newly diagnosed coeliacs start on a gluten-free diet by not eating the products that obviously contain gluten – anything with wheat, barley, rye and oats. That's a great step, but sometimes hidden amounts of gluten are still being eaten. It is up to every coeliac to research everything that goes into their mouths. If you're not getting better, often it's because there is still some gluten left in your diet.

First, recheck all the labels of any product you're eating. If nothing looks suspect, then ask yourself the following questions.

- Am I eating butter or margarine that may have breadcrumbs from wheat bread in it?
- Am I toasting gluten-free bread in a toaster that has had wheat bread toasted in it?
- Does my kitchen worktop have on it traces of anything that is made with gluten that might be able to get into my food?
- Is my breadboard clean, free of any wheat bread crumbs?
- Are my cosmetics gluten-free?
- Are my medicines – over-the-counter and prescription ones – gluten-free?
- Am I eating fried foods from restaurants where they fry their food in the same oil as breaded foods?

- Are you kneading wholemeal bread, pizza bases or other dough, pastry, say, for the family?

Some of these questions may sound ridiculous, but gluten is everywhere and some coeliacs react to even minute traces of gluten. You really must look at everything and question whether or not it is gluten-free. In the beginning this may seem like a monumental task, but soon you will learn what you can and cannot have and to follow your instincts.

Food intolerances

If you're still feeling bad on a gluten-free diet another possibility is that you have one or more food intolerances. The most common food intolerance for coeliacs is of lactose, which usually goes away after you eliminate it for six months and are on a gluten-free diet.

An easy way to find out if you have an intolerance of a specific food is to keep a food diary. Write down everything you eat and the day and time you eat it. Also, write down any physical symptoms you experience, again noting the time and date. After one week, look back at your diary and see if you can spot any relationship between a food you ate and a physical symptom. For example, if you ate gluten-free ice-cream and 30 minutes later you had diarrhoea, you might suspect you have an allergy to dairy products. Eliminate dairy foods for one week and note if your physical health has improved. Then, eat some dairy foods and record how you feel. If you are intolerant of them, you could have a reaction any time from immediately after you ate them to 24–48 hours later, so beware. An elimination diet like this is a helpful method to use for any food you suspect is making you feel ill.

Go to your doctor

If you have tried the above and still not identified why you're feeling bad, go to your doctor. Your doctor can do more tests and help you identify the source of the problem.

6

Living in a gluten-free world

Jumping over hurdles

You're at the starting line, preparing to jump over hurdles, visualizing the satisfaction of jumping over every hurdle without stumbling and making it to the finish line successfully, perhaps in record time. When you get to the finish line you'll feel good. You can see the end, but know that each hurdle is potentially dangerous. There are hecklers in the crowd who watch your every move like hawks. You know what you have to do to get to the end, but some days you will be able to jump better than others.

On a gluten-free diet, you will have many hurdles to jump over. They do not have to be painful, but you must be prepared to deal with them if you're going to achieve your goal of staying on a gluten-free diet. Each person will be able to jump over the hurdles at a different pace and level of comfort. Go at your own pace, always honouring your unique needs.

This chapter presents six hurdles you will face, giving you strategies for jumping over them with ease. If you pace yourself to jump over each hurdle, you will get to the end and achieve your goal of living in a gluten-free world.

Hurdle 1: having a positive attitude

If you're going to stay on a gluten-free diet, you must begin with a positive attitude. You can do it. Believing you can stay gluten-free is half the battle to living in a gluten-free world. Your mind is a powerful tool. It will be able to get you through situations that appear tough on the surface, but underneath are not that difficult.

As you start your gluten-free diet, take a moment to ask yourself the following.

- How do I feel now?
- How do I want to feel?

Write your answers down somewhere and go back to them periodically to give yourself the motivation you may need at times to stay on the diet. After a month on the diet, ask yourself one more question.

- How does a gluten-free diet make me feel?

Once you see the change in your health, you will be convinced that living in a gluten-free world is worth it.

Hurdle 2: preparing your family and friends

The foods you can and cannot eat are shocking to many people, and your family and friends are no exception. As they are often the people you surround yourself with, they are your support network. If they reject, laugh at or insult your diet, this may affect your ability to stay on it. Their support is crucial. Without it, you may begin to 'just cheat occasionally'. Friends and relatives may not realize how important it is for them to offer encouragement.

Most family and friends will take your diet seriously if you take it seriously. Being serious about eating a gluten-free diet does not mean you should walk around with a stern face and lecture everyone about your dietary requirements. On the contrary, laugh with your family and friends, tell jokes about the foods you eat, but don't begin to cheat here and there, because no one will take your diet seriously if you cheat.

Providing them with information

The people you eat with every day are the first you must educate about your diet. They cannot understand your diet and provide support for you if you do not explain why you are eating gluten-free foods. There are several ways in which you could do this.

- *Write something on coeliac disease* and a gluten-free diet to hand out. A simple, one-page explanation can provide all the information people need without your having to repeat again and again why you're eating what you're eating. You could photocopy information you think might be useful for people to know or get creative and write a coeliac factsheet, devising a simple crossword puzzle at the bottom to test family and friends on their knowledge!
- *Have a gluten-free dinner party* Many of your friends and family may only have vague ideas about what a gluten-free diet is, but seeing and tasting gluten-free foods will show them just how simple cooking a gluten-free meal can be. A dinner party can be an easy, fun way to introduce gluten-free cooking to the people you care about. To facilitate a discussion on coeliac disease and the diet, you could put an index card in front of everyone's table setting with a fact about coeliac disease you think they should

know. For example, on one side write, 'What is gluten?' and on the other side answer the question. Then let everyone share the information they have received. Don't force people to share – many times one person will read out the information on their card and the conversation will just take off from there. Other topics you could put on index cards include 'Foods to avoid on a gluten-free diet', 'The history of coeliac disease', 'What is coeliac disease?' Use your imagination and think of your own!

- *Organize a gluten-free scavenger hunt* This is great to do with a family, especially children, to educate everyone on the foods coeliacs can eat. You can have a scavenger hunt inside the home or out. Here's how.
- In preparation, assemble at least ten products that are gluten-free and ten that are not gluten-free. If the ingredients are not obvious (like bread), then write out the ingredients of the product and attach this label to the product. This will teach everyone to read ingredients – a very important skill for anyone who is going to live with or cook for a coeliac.
- Write a list of all the gluten-free products each participant needs to find.
- Hide all the products – gluten-free and not gluten-free – throughout the area you have designated for the scavenger hunt.
- Instruct each participant to search for the gluten-free items, warning them that there are also items with gluten hidden in the area, but to only collect the ones that are gluten-free.
- The first person to find the most gluten-free items wins.
- Give them a prize – maybe some gluten-free biscuits!

Hurdle 3: shopping for gluten-free foods

There are a lot of foods to eat that have no gluten in them. Shopping for food on a gluten-free diet may initially seem impossible, but you will soon get used to it. The key things to do are to ask questions if you're not sure whether or not something is gluten-free and to always read labels. The food list produced by The Coeliac Society is the most reliable information currently available in the UK for coeliacs, so it is worth getting hold of a copy (see Useful addresses at the end of the book).

Food on prescription

Once you are officially diagnosed as a coeliac, you can order gluten-free foods by prescription from your local chemist. The list of prescription foods includes gluten-free breads, pasta, biscuits and other products that will assist you in living on a gluten-free diet. Consult The Coeliac Society's magazine *The Crossed Grain* and its food list for a list of what items are available on prescription.

Consider yourself lucky; for the cost of a prescription, you can often get many gluten-free products through the National Health Service. This is not the case for many coeliacs in other parts of the world, who have to buy all their special diet foods themselves.

You are not exempt from prescription charges because you have coeliac disease, as the DSS does not consider the condition a chronically sick disorder. However, you might be exempt if you are under 16, in receipt of a state retirement pension or have an exemption certificate for a specific reason other than coeliac disease (such as you would during pregnancy). Anyone above the age of 16 may also be exempt on grounds of low income. If you fall into any of these categories, go into your local Social Security office and ask for details.

If you are not exempt, it may be best for you to use the 'Season Ticket' facility. Once you purchase this annually, you do not have to pay anything when you fill out any prescription for that year. It's good value for money if you're likely to get many gluten-free products on prescription.

Healthfood shops

You may initially want to visit a healthfood shop to see what gluten-free products they offer. While many coeliacs find that it is not necessary to buy a lot of products from a healthfood shop, it is a good idea to familiarize yourself with what they offer. Before you go though, think about what information you want to get out of the trip. What types of gluten-free products are you looking for? Bring a summary of what a gluten-free diet is with you, in case the salesperson doesn't know. Ask the salesperson to assist you in your search.

Healthfood shops are usually very useful places to buy gluten-free flours not available in the supermarkets. They often stock other gluten-free products, too, which you may be interested in if you can't get them on prescription.

Supermarkets

Supermarkets are where most people do their shopping, but now when you go you'll have to adjust your way of thinking. You can no longer fling something into your trolley on a whim and devour it when you get home. Whenever you pick up any product you must *think coeliac*. This means reading labels, checking your Coeliac Society food list, rechecking every ingredient that's going to enter your body before you even think of eating it. You must be meticulous and serious about this endeavour because gluten will initially seem like it's everywhere. If you *think coeliac* before you buy any product, then you're on your way to living gluten-free.

To make the supermarket your friend, not foe, make a food list before you start shopping. Once you've identified what foods you want to purchase, see which ones are gluten-free. Whichever foods are not gluten-free, try to think of a substitute that might be very similar to the product you want. Maybe the can of soup you usually buy is not gluten-free. If you cannot find another soup that is gluten-free, buy the ingredients for a simple home-made soup. Then spend part of your day off making a couple of home-made gluten-free soups and freeze them. Home-made soups are usually much nicer than canned soups anyway and not very difficult to make.

Share your supermarket burden with those you live with. Take them along to the supermarket and show them what to look for when they're reading labels so they will notice an ingredient with gluten in it. Let them shop for you sometimes, and see how they do!

In the beginning, you will find that it will take longer to do your shopping than it used to, but after a few months, once you're into *think coeliac* mode, you will find you're over that hurdle and it gets easier and easier to go food shopping.

Hurdle 4: going on holiday

Your diet should not stop you from going on holiday and, indeed, many coeliacs are able to maintain their gluten-free diet while on holiday. It may be frustrating in the beginning, but, with a positive attitude, if you want to travel you can. The list below will help you prepare yourself for going on holiday.

- *Always carry snacks* If you're hungry and cannot find anything gluten-free, you may panic and eat anything to stave off the hunger. Make sure you have provisions that could get you through at least 24 hours. Rice cakes are a great option because they're light to carry and easy to eat with cheese or meat. Also, gluten-free bread travels well if it is sealed in its packet.
- *Call the hotel to explain your condition* Many good hotels will be able to understand your needs and cater to them. When you arrive at the hotel you should speak to the head chef to remind him or

her how crucial it is that your food is gluten-free, making it clear that you could be very sick if you ingest gluten. Don't assume they'll remember you're gluten-free, and speak up if you think the food may not be gluten-free. As before, if you take the diet seriously, so will they.

- *Get an advice sheet from The Coeliac Society* These sheets are available for many countries and offer hints on travel and translations of useful phrases for the country you're visiting. They have a leaflet on airline meals, a brief catering guide and a concise explanation of coeliac disease, too.
- *Go into healthfood shops* Many countries sell gluten-free products in healthfood shops. It's good to locate a shop like this because you may be able to pick up an extra loaf of gluten-free bread or biscuits for your journey.
- *Try a self-catering holiday* Many coeliacs feel more comfortable making their own food on holiday so they know what they're eating. There are many options for self-catering throughout the world – renting a villa, a seaside cottage or a ski house are all fun options. Depending on where you're going, you may have to take many of your gluten-free provisions with you, so make sure you've packed enough food with you to last the whole holiday!
- *Bring gluten-free flour* If you are abroad for a long time, you could approach a local baker and ask if they'll bake some gluten-free loaves for you. Many bakers will, so don't be shy. Make sure you explain your diet and ask them to bake the loaves in an area of the bakery where no gluten has been.
- *Order a special meal on airplanes* Airline meals are often a source of great frustration for coeliacs. Your best approach would be to first ask for a gluten-free meal when you buy your ticket. If the booking agent does not find that such a meal is available, then ask for an Asian, vegetarian meal, which is usually gluten-free, or a fruit platter, so at least you have something you can eat. You should also always travel with your own stash of gluten-free provisions.
- *If you become ill* As coeliac disease is not common, if you fall sick, it is best to request a paediatrician (children's doctor) who will most likely have heard of coeliac disease because it is more commonly diagnosed in children than adults. This doctor may then be able to refer you to an adult coeliac specialist. If this is not possible, make sure any doctor treating you has been informed of your condition.

- *Have a sense of humour* There will be moments, such as when the food you ordered at your hotel arrives with a heavy sauce full of gluten, that you'll want to scream with frustration. When this happens, instead, take a deep breath, and laugh. Laughter and a good sense of humour while travelling will get you through a lot of ups and downs.

Hurdle 5: eating out

After the shock wears off about changing your diet, you are going to have to face the reality that sometimes you will be eating out of your home. You might want to take some time to adjust to your new diet at home for a while, declining dinner invitations or work events, but, eventually, you will no doubt feel the desire to socialize again. When you do, arm yourself with some of the coping techniques below.

Dinner parties

Are you frightened of showing up at a dinner party because there won't be anything to eat for you? This doesn't have to be the case. Tell the person who invited you about your food requirements and make sure they understand how important it is that you not eat any gluten. Most hosts will be happy you told them and try to accommodate your needs. Suggest something simple they could prepare for you or offer to contribute a gluten-free dish to the meal. You may feel initially like you're being fussy, but you have to eat.

If you're going somewhere and you don't think there'll be many gluten-free options, make sure you eat something before you go. There is nothing worse than watching everyone else eat while you starve. Also, bring a snack with you, like a banana or some gluten-free biscuits. If someone makes a comment about your 'strange eating habits', explain you're a coeliac. Most people will accept this and be interested in your condition.

Those who do not accept your diet usually react in this way because in almost every culture we are socialized to believe certain foods are 'normal' and as some of your gluten-free foods may not fall into that category, some people will feel uncomfortable with, for example, you eating gluten-free biscuits at a dinner party, viewing your food as abnormal. This can be very aggravating and intimidating for many coeliacs, but when you meet this sort of person, it's best to show compassion, as they do not accept your diet because they are victims of society's pressure to make people conform to only one way of thinking. 'Normal' and 'abnormal' food is only relative to one's experience. Many people in other cultures would think it completely abnormal to be eating cold, processed cereals out of boxes every morning and putting vinegar on chips. Vegetarianism was also considered abnormal in our own culture until fairly recently. If your food makes you healthy, then ignore the culture mongers who laugh at foods that are different from their own. Their reaction is more a reflection on them than you.

Restaurants

Eating in restaurants can be challenging, but not impossible. Calling the restaurant in advance to speak to the chef is usually the best approach. It's best to call at least 24 hours before you are going to arrive, so the chef can have enough time to prepare your meal, and to call in the morning when the chef is not too busy.

If you don't feel comfortable doing this or have decided to go to a restaurant on impulse, so there is no time to check with the chef in advance, here's a quick guide to what you can eat to get you through the menu.

- *Cocktails* Most wines, tequila and rums are OK to drink. Avoid any grain-based alcohol, like beer or vodka.
- *Starters* Choose any fresh fruit, Parma ham and melon. Avoid most soups (you just can't be sure what's in them), pâtés, anything with mayonnaise, fish cocktails.
- *Main courses* Try plain, grilled meats, plain omelettes, plain vegetables with butter. Stay away from anything with stuffing, gravy, sauces, dressings or fried foods cooked in the same oil as breaded foods.
- *Desserts* Fresh fruit is the safest option. Dairy cream is also safe. Avoid ice-cream, puddings, pies, ice-cream wafers. While some may be OK to eat if they're the right brand, you cannot be certain in a restaurant what you're eating.
- *After dinner drinks* Freshly ground coffee and tea with milk are safe. All sherry, wine, champagne, whisky and brandy are OK to drink.

The golden rule is if you're not sure what the ingredients in your meal are, ask. If the chef (not the waiter) cannot guarantee that it's gluten-free, then don't eat it.

To save yourself a lot of worry, try to find a couple of restaurants near where you live or work that can cater to your gluten-free needs. These will be your 'safe' restaurants, so when someone suggests going out to eat you can suggest a restaurant with little fear that you'll get sick. Once you find a 'safe' restaurant, where you develop a rapport with the chef and waiting staff so they know your needs, the hassles of eating out will lessen.

Work

To eat or not to eat? That is the question for many coeliacs when they start a gluten-free diet and are confronted with lunchtime at work. Pulling out your gluten-free bread and biscuits while the rest of your fellow workers are eating their sandwiches can be embarrassing at first. Many of them will surely have questions, some will laugh, others will ask lots of questions about the diet. All of this can seem quite overwhelming when you're trying to adjust to the diet yourself. Don't despair, you can eat at work if you're prepared to forget about what people think and do a little planning beforehand.

Bring your own food to work. Preparing some food the night before and putting it into a suitable plastic container is not very difficult once you get use to it. You could make a bit more of your evening meal and save the leftovers for lunch the next day or combine these with something different. For example, you could cook extra gluten-free pasta, put some on the side and mix it with tuna the next day for lunch. You could make a sandwich with gluten-free bread, bring gluten-free biscuits or bananas as snacks or bake a potato the night before and eat it with a gluten-free topping. If you plan ahead, you don't have to be faced with running out of the office for something only to find that there's nothing you can eat.

Going out for lunch is not impossible either. See under Restaurants above for some ideas.

In hospital

If you have to go into hospital, make sure staff know you require a gluten-free diet before you are admitted. Some hospitals are quite good at catering for this diet; others are not. Ask to speak to the hospital dietitian to explain your needs because they are usually the most informed about special diets and what that particular hospital can offer. When you check in, remind staff that you need gluten-free meals.

Even with all this checking, it is best to also take an assortment of gluten-free products with you when you are in hospital, just to be sure you have food. Many coeliacs have complained that their so-called gluten-free meals were not gluten-free. As hospitals don't regularly cater for coeliacs (as opposed to diabetics), they may not get it right all the time. You know what you can and cannot eat, so you must be the final judge of whether something is gluten-free or not. Don't eat anything that looks questionable.

If you're really dissatisfied, write the hospital a friendly note explaining how your needs were not met. Don't just complain verbally, put it in writing! The more coeliacs speak up and inform hospitals that their meals are not meeting gluten-free standards, the better it will be for coeliacs in the future.

Hurdle 6: eating at home

Eating at home, while much easier than eating out, still requires thought and planning when you are just starting. You must think about what ingredients you are using in everything you make, consider where gluten may be hiding in your kitchen, possibly contaminating gluten-free food, and may have to juggle cooking gluten-free meals for yourself and another meal for the rest of your family, as they can eat gluten. It's not such a large task, but it does need to be taken seriously. Below are some hints on how to start thinking gluten-free at home.

Preparing your kitchen

If you think you're completely safe from gluten at home, think again. As even a minute amount of gluten can cause damage to the lining of the small intestine in some coeliacs, you must prepare your kitchen so it is totally gluten-free. Here's how.

- *Mark a set of kitchen equipment to be used exclusively for gluten-free foods* This will decrease the risk that kitchen equipment may not be washed sufficiently to avoid them contaminating your gluten-free foods. Wooden spoons and chopping boards are ideal places for such food residues to hide in, for example. It is highly recommended that you use a coloured marker or stickers (anything that stands out) to indicate what equipment is gluten-free so no one you're living with will use yours by mistake. A mark can be scratched onto baking tins with a file so they can be set aside for you.
- *Cook gluten-free foods first* If you're cooking a meal with gluten-free foods and foods with gluten, make the gluten-free foods first because, if the kitchen is clean, you can then be sure the food you prepare will be free of any gluten.
- *If you wear an apron, use one that only you wear* because if you share aprons, the person using the apron before you could have made something with gluten and wiped their hands on the apron

71

and you could then find this is a source of contamination of your food.

- *Wash your hands well before you start cooking* Make sure your hands are extra clean, even under the fingernails! Gluten can hide anywhere.
- *Always clean up well* and encourage the people you live with to clean up well after cooking any food. This will ensure that your food isn't accidentally contaminated with gluten.
- *Keep gluten-free products in their own containers* and, preferably, in a cupboard on their own. This will ensure there is no confusion about what is gluten-free and what's not.

The next step in preparing your kitchen is to consider what equipment you should have to assist you in making gluten-free products. Think about your needs and decide what equipment is essential for you. Most coeliacs find they use the following equipment frequently:

- grain mill
- food processor
- pressure cooker
- breadmaker.

The benefits of these four pieces of equipment far outweigh their cost. They will mean preparing your food will take less time and be more enjoyable. A *grain mill* grinds whole seeds into flour so you can be sure that there is no possibility of gluten contamination, which can happen in commercial mills. A *food processor* is an excellent way to purée or blend fresh foods quickly that are difficult to mix by hand. In addition, a *pressure cooker* saves you time and allows you to cook from scratch, very helpful for coeliacs. Finally, a *breadmaker*, while not essential and quite expensive, can open up an entirely new dimension to eating gluten-free bread. It is no hassle to make your own bread and it tastes good too!

Meal planning

Not everyone's a planner. Whether you are or not, you may want to plan your meals for the first few weeks on a gluten-free diet to give yourself an idea of what foods you can eat.

To plan meals that are right for you, take out a pen and paper and ask yourself, 'What were typical breakfasts, lunches and evening meals for me before I was diagnosed?' You could put the headings

'Breakfast', 'Lunch' and so on across the top of a sheet of paper and include a 'Snack' heading, too, if you like to snack.

Look at your lists and circle which items are not gluten-free. Then use a clean sheet of paper to compose your new, gluten-free diet for five days, using the same headings. You may want to refer back to Chapter 5 to check what foods you can eat. Also, look again at your lists of circled items to note which foods you will no longer be able to have in your diet. You could substitute similar gluten-free versions of these things – say, make a gravy with cornflour instead of wheat flour – or you could be more original and create your own dishes. The lists below will help give you some ideas for simple gluten-free meals you could use to start yourself off on the diet.

Breakfast

Eggs with gluten-free toast
Corn-based breakfast cereals and milk
Grilled bacon
Fried potatoes

Lunch

Canned salmon, tuna or sardines (in brine or oil, not a sauce)
Jacket potato
Fresh salads
Sandwiches made using gluten-free bread and fresh meat or cheese

Evening meals

Grilled meats and fish
Vegetables cooked in a gluten-free sauce
Gluten-free gravy
Rice

Desserts

Fresh fruit
Gluten-free biscuits

Snacks

Fresh fruit
Popcorn
Raw vegetable sticks
Toasted sunflower seeds

You should always have a supply of staples in the house. These include rice, potatoes, pulses, gluten-free pasta, gluten-free flours and gluten-free biscuits. In an emergency, these foods will allow you to create a meal that's gluten-free and, with a few spices and herbs, one that is tasty, too.

Make simple meals to begin with and then, once you've been on the diet for a while, experiment with more elaborate dishes. However, remember, the more complicated the dish, the more you must keep track of all the ingredients you're using. Gluten-free cooking is easy if you keep it simple.

Meals for children

If you believe your child can stay on the diet, this positive attitude will rub off on them. Gluten-free foods can be fun for kids and don't have to be seen as a pain. Many of the foods mentioned above can also be served to children. Try to make the food colourful and attractive, while providing a nutritious meal.

Children's parties can be a bit more challenging, but not impossible. If your child is invited to a party, offer to bring a dish to the party that your child can eat and other children would enjoy. If you are organizing a party at home, make gluten-free treats for everyone, such as:

- cheeses
- home-made sausage rolls
- home-made beef or chicken burgers
- jacket potatoes
- fresh fruit
- baked bananas
- gluten-free ice-cream
- home-made gluten-free biscuits and cakes.

A coeliac child needs to be encouraged and supported to stay on a gluten-free diet. This means not tempting your child by keeping lots of food items with gluten in the house. Also, make meals for the whole family that are gluten-free and then let those who can eat gluten add ordinary bread or gravy. Your child will feel a lot more normal about the diet if you act as if it were normal.

Scrapes, bumps and bruises

Now that you've jumped over all the hurdles, it's time to forget about your scrapes, bumps and bruises and start cooking. The next chapter is full of gluten-free recipes that even a novice cook will be able to make.

7
Gluten-free cooking

This chapter provides recipes to get you started on a gluten-free diet. These are just a few of the recipes that you can make on a gluten-free diet. If you enjoy cooking, there are plenty of gluten-free cookery books in the bookshops that will give you a more complete range of the meals you could make.

BREADS

Thought you couldn't live without bread? You don't have to. Have a go at making your own gluten-free bread.

Gluten-free Flour Mix

This mix can be used for all recipes that use flour. If you prefer not to make your own, commercial gluten-free flour mixes are readily available.

> *350 g (12 oz) rice flour (white or brown rice)*
> *100 g (4 oz) potato flour*
> *75 g (3 oz) soya flour (omit if you cannot tolerate it)*

Mix well and store in the refrigerator or freezer in an airtight container.

Quick Gluten-free Breads

550 g (1¼ lbs) rice flour (white
 or brown rice)
175 g (6 oz) cornflour
3 tablespoons mashed potatoes
3 teaspoons gluten-free baking
 powder
2 tablespoons unflavoured
 gelatin

1 teaspoon salt
100 g (4 oz) sugar or honey
3 eggs
300 ml (10 fl oz) buttermilk
40 ml (2 fl oz) corn oil or
 melted margarine
225 g (8 oz) cottage cheese

Preheat the oven to 190°C/375°F/Gas 5. Grease two 450g (1 lb) loaf
tins. Mix the flours, potatoes, baking powder, gelatin, salt and sugar or
honey together. Then add the remaining ingredients and mix together
until creamy. As this is not a yeasted bread, it can be baked
immediately. Divide the mixture between the prepared loaf tins and
bake in the preheated oven for 55 minutes. They are done when, if you
turn them out of their tins, they sound hollow when you tap them on
the bottom. If they are not done, let them bake 5 to 10 minutes longer.

Variations
To make raisin bread, add 225 g (8 oz) of raisins and 1 teaspoon of
ground cinnamon. For fruit bread, add 225 g (8 oz) chopped dried
apricots or dates, plus 225 g (8 oz) chopped nuts. For banana bread,
add 450 g (1 lb) mashed bananas, 1 extra egg and 1 extra teaspoon of
baking powder.

Rice Bread

100 g (4 oz) grated carrot
1 egg
150 ml (5 fl oz) milk or water,
* if you're lactose intolerant*
100 g (4 oz) rice flour

100 g (4 oz) potato flour
25 g (1 oz) soya flour
1 teaspoon bicarbonate of soda
2 tablespoons corn oil
1 teaspoon sugar

Preheat the oven to 220°C/425°F/Gas 7. Purée the carrots, egg and milk together. Mix together all the dry ingredients with the oil. Gently fold the flour mixture into the carrrot purée until just mixed. (Don't overmix and do not leave to stand as the light structure of the bread dough will be lost.) Pour the batter 2.5 cm (1 in) deep into a shallow, 25 cm (10 in) square baking tray. Bake in the preheated oven for 35–40 minutes. The loaf is done when if you poke a skewer into the bread it comes out clean.

Variations
Instead of the carrots, try adding your favourite fruit (bananas and apples work well) or 100 g (4 oz) of chestnuts or tofu!

Cornbread

225 g (8 oz) yellow cornmeal
225 g (8 oz) rice flour
50 g (2 oz) sugar
4 teaspoons bicarbonate
  of soda

½ teaspoon salt
250 ml (8 fl oz) buttermilk
1 egg
50 ml (2 fl oz) corn oil

Preheat the oven to 220°C/425°F/Gas 7. Grease a 20 cm (8 in) square baking tin. Mix all the dry ingredients together. Add the buttermilk, egg and oil. Beat well for a couple of minutes then pour the mixture into the prepared baking tin and bake in the preheated oven for 20 minutes. It is done when, if the baking tin is removed, it sounds hollow when tapped on the bottom. Allow to bake longer if not done.

Variations
Add 100 g (4 oz) finely chopped onion to the batter and sprinkle Cheddar cheese on top. Add to the batter 175 g (6 oz) of crispy, crumbled bacon. Try adding 1½ tablespoons of deseeded and finely chopped fresh green chilli to the batter.

SAUCES

You can have gravy and white sauce, just not thickened with white or wholemeal wheat flour. Try these and spot the difference!

White Sauce

25 g (1 oz) cornflour
300 ml (10 fl oz) milk
salt and freshly ground black pepper

Mix the cornflour and a little of the milk together to form a paste. Gradually, little by little, stir in the remaining milk. Slowly heat the sauce until it is simmering, stirring continuously. Gently simmer for 5 minutes until it has thickened.

Variations
Try adding 120 ml (4 fl oz) of tahini, for a rich, sesame sauce. Chop and then fry one onion and stir it into the cooked sauce. A cheese sauce is nice. To make one, just add 100 g (4 oz) grated cheese to the cooked sauce and stir until it has melted and is smooth.

Gravy

300 ml (10 fl oz) juice from roasted meat or vegetables
1 teaspoon cornflour
salt and freshly ground black pepper

Spoon the fat off the juice. Allow the remaining juice to cool. Mix the cornflour into a paste with a little cold water in a saucepan. Over a medium heat, slowly add the juice to the cornflour paste, stirring continuously. Simmer the gravy for 5 minutes. Add salt and pepper to taste.

Variations
Add one chopped and then fried onion.

Peanut Sauce

100 g (4 oz) peanut butter
120 ml (4 fl oz) milk

Blend the ingredients together until smooth.

Variations
Use tahini instead of the peanut butter, when you want a sesame flavour. Use soya milk instead of dairy milk.

SALAD DRESSINGS

Bought salad dressings are risky, so make your own to be sure it's gluten-free!

Lemon Herbed Dressing

$\frac{1}{2}$ lemon
1 teaspoon fresh rosemary
120 ml (4 fl oz) olive oil
salt and freshly ground black pepper

Squeeze the juice from the lemon into the olive oil and mix them together thoroughly (a screw-topped jar is good for this). Chop the rosemary and add to the lemon juice and olive oil mixture. Add salt and pepper to taste. Shake well before serving.

Variations
Add any combination of herbs you like.

Honey Mustard Dressing

> 120 ml (4 fl oz) olive oil
> 1 teaspoon mustard
> 1 teaspoon honey

Put all the ingredients into a clean, screw-topped jar and shake to mix them together thoroughly. Shake well before serving.

Variations
Add herbs of your choice. Substitute any sweetener for the honey.

SOUPS

Soups are great meals, on their own or with your own choice of accompaniments. If you make soup and freeze it in small containers, you'll always have something to eat when you don't feel like cooking.

Root Vegetable Soup

This is one of the easiest soups in the world to make, especially if you have a blender or food processor.

3 carrots, peeled
2 turnips, peeled
1 onion, peeled
2 tablespoons olive oil

piece of fresh root ginger the
   size of your thumb
$1\frac{1}{2}$ teaspoons fresh rosemary

Put all the ingredients in a pan, pour in enough water to cover and bring to the boil. Simmer for 20 minutes (or pressure cook for 8 minutes), or until the vegetables are tender, adding more water if necessary. Pour the soup into a blender or food processor and blend until the soup is your favourite consistency, then serve. (If you don't have a blender or food processor, mash the vegetables with a masher.)

Variations
Use different root vegetables, like swedes. Don't use any oil. Use different herbs and spices to flavour the soup.

Creamy Courgette Soup

1 onion, chopped
1–2 tablespoons vegetable oil
4–5 courgettes, chopped

3 potatoes, peeled and chopped
salt and freshly ground black
  pepper to taste

Fry the onion in the oil until it has browned. Add the courgettes and potatoes, pour in enough water to cover. Add salt and pepper to taste, then bring to the boil. Simmer for 20 minutes. Use a blender or food processor or masher to purée the soup, then serve.

Variations
For a creamy soup with oats instead of potatoes, add 100 g (4 oz) of oats in at the same time as you add the courgettes and water and stir constantly until boiling. Substitute any other vegetable for the courgettes, such as broccoli.

Lentil Soup

225 g (8 oz) green lentils
1.2 litres (2 pints) water
1 onion, chopped

1 garlic clove, crushed
1 teaspoon root ginger, crushed
50 ml (2 fl oz) olive oil

Bring the lentils to the boil in the water. Simmer for 45 minutes. Meanwhile, fry the onion, garlic and ginger together in the oil until they have softened. Add this mixture to the lentils 10 minutes before the end of cooking.

Variations
Add gluten-free fried bacon bits to the lentils. Use red lentils instead of green if you're in a hurry as these cook in only 20–25 minutes.

MAIN DISHES

There are many main dishes that are gluten-free, so you shouldn't have many problems thinking of something to cook. If there are ingredients in these recipes that you cannot tolerate at the moment, read the variations and try to think of a substitute – none of the recipes are carved in stone! You are free to change any recipe to suit your needs.

Soy Chicken

50 ml (2 fl oz) corn oil
3 tablespoons gluten-free
  Bragg soy sauce or tamari
1 teaspoon salt
1 teaspoon gluten-free curry
  powder

4 boneless, skinless chicken
  breasts
1 onion, thinly sliced
3 medium tomatoes, chopped
1 teaspoon grated root ginger
2 garlic cloves, chopped

Preheat the oven to 190°C/375°F/Gas 5. Put the oil, soy sauce or tamari, salt and curry powder into a bowl and mix together well. Coat the chicken breasts with this mixture and place them in a baking dish. Sprinkle the onion slices, tomatoes, ginger and garlic all over the chicken breasts. Bake in the preheated oven for 25–30 minutes, checking them periodically and basting if they start to get dry.

Potato and Ham Bake

750 g (1½ lbs) potatoes,
  peeled and sliced
2 tablespoons vegetable oil
1 teaspoon paprika
50 ml (2 fl oz) milk
450 g (1 lb) gluten-free ham,
  diced
1 onion, diced

¼ green pepper, diced
450 g (1 lb) sharp Cheddar
  cheese, grated
6 eggs
50 g (2 oz) sour cream
salt and freshly ground black
  pepper

Preheat the oven to 200°C/400°F/Gas 6. Fry the potato slices in the oil, paprika and milk until golden brown. Layer the fried potatoes, ham, onion, green pepper and cheese in an oiled 20-cm (8-in) square baking dish or tin. Mix together the remaining ingredients and pour over the layered ingredients in the baking dish or tin. Bake in the preheated oven for 55 minutes, until meltingly tender.

Variations
Use turkey instead of ham. Don't use any meat and you have a great vegetarian dish. Add the herbs of your choice.

Nutloaf

225 g (8 oz) onion, chopped
2 garlic cloves, crushed
2 tablespoons vegetable oil
225 g (8 oz) hazelnuts,
  chopped
150 g (5 oz) gluten-free
  breadcrumbs

2 eggs
150 ml (5 fl oz) water
1 teaspoon fresh rosemary
salt and freshly ground black
  pepper

Preheat the oven to 200°C/400°F/Gas 6. Fry the onion and garlic in the oil until they have softened. In a food processor, mix the nuts and breadcrumbs together. Transfer the nut and breadcrumb mixture to a bowl, add the onion and garlic mixture and mix by hand. Beat the eggs, water and rosemary into the mixture and season to taste with salt and pepper. Place the mixture in a greased and lined 450 g (1 lb) loaf tin and bake in the preheated oven for 50–60 minutes.

Variations
Add any combination of herbs you like. Use milk (or soya milk) instead of water, for a richer flavour. Substitute walnuts for the hazelnuts.

Tim's Groundnut Stew

5 tablespoons vegetable oil
(peanut oil is best for this)
2 large onions, sliced or
chopped
2 garlic cloves, chopped or
crushed
2 fresh hot chillies, chopped,
or ground hot dried red
peppers, optional
25 g (1 oz) fresh root ginger,
peeled and grated
1 teaspoon whole cumin seeds,
optional
4 large fresh tomatoes, peeled
and roughly chopped, or
400 g (14 oz) tinned peeled
tomatoes, roughly chopped
4 medium potatoes, peeled and
quartered

2 large carrots, peeled and
chopped
2 teaspoons tomato purée or
2 more chopped, peeled
tomatoes
450 g (1 lb) cooked chickpeas
or other bean (but not kidney
beans) or meat of your
choice
1 teaspoon fresh thyme or
mixed herbs
2 bay leaves, optional
salt and freshly ground black
pepper
4 heaped tablespoons peanut
butter (sugar-free is best)

Fry the onions in the hot oil in a large saucepan until they are just starting to turn brown. Add the garlic, chillies and ginger and stir-fry for 1 minute. Add the cumin seeds and stir for another minute. (If you are using meat, then add the meat now and fry for a minute or 2, stirring all the time.) Add the tomatoes, stir to make sure nothing is sticking to the bottom of the pan and bring to the boil. Add the potatoes and carrots and simmer, covered, for 10–15 minutes. Check towards the end of this time and add a little extra water if necessary. (If you are using meat, then increase the cooking time to allow the meat to cook right through and do not add the potatoes until after the meat is done, otherwise they will overcook and break up into the stew.) Add the tomato purée or extra tomatoes, chickpeas or beans, herbs, bay leaves and salt and pepper to taste, stirring them all in. Simmer for 10 more minutes, adding a little extra water if necessary (the potatoes, chickpeas or beans and other ingredients should be almost covered by the juice). Add the peanut butter, stirring it in thoroughly. Then, cook for about 5–15 minutes more, or until the potatoes are done – the exact time this takes depends on the variety of potatoes used.

Variations
Use any vegetables you like. Courgettes and squash taste nice in this dish. Add shelled hard-boiled eggs (one per person) 10 minutes before serving. Add more chillies if you like it hot! You can substitute meat for the chickpeas or beans – just follow the instructions in brackets in the method.

Flourless Pancakes

225 g (8 oz) cooked brown rice
1 egg
120 ml (4 fl oz) milk
50 g (2 oz) cheese, diced
1 tablespoon oil

Process the rice, egg and milk together in a blender or food processor for 1 minute, until you have a smooth purée. Add the cheese and process for 15 more seconds. The mixture will now be lumpy. Heat a little oil in a frying pan, pour in 50 ml (2 fl oz) of batter and cook the pancake until it is golden brown on both sides. Repeat until you have used up all the batter.

Variations
Leave out the cheese and, after the pancakes are cooked, top with maple syrup for sweet rather than savoury pancakes.

CREATIVE SIDE DISHES

Gluten-free side dishes don't have to mean boiled potatoes with no gravy. Try making one of the following quick and easy creative side dishes to make your food look and taste better.

Baked Squash

Squashes taste great and, although they're not commonly served in Britain, most major supermarkets sell them in season.

> *1 small cooking squash (acorn or butternut are best)*
> *250 ml (8 fl oz) water*
> *1–2 tablespoons olive oil*
> *salt and freshly ground black pepper*

Preheat the oven to 200°C/400°F/Gas 6. Cut the squash into quarters, lenghthwise. Scoop out the seeds and discard. Place the pieces of squash in a lightly oiled baking tin or dish, skin side down, cut side up and pour the water around them. Cover the tin or dish with oiled foil, placing it oiled side down. Bake in the preheated oven for about 1 hour, until the flesh is tender. Then, take the tin or dish out of the oven and brush the pieces of squash with a little oil, season with salt and pepper to taste and serve.

Variations
Use butter or margarine instead of oil. Sprinkle finely chopped or crushed garlic over the pieces of squash before baking. Try sprinkling nutmeg and cinnamon over the baked squash.

Sesame Broccoli

2–3 tablespoons sesame seeds
2 heads fresh broccoli, chopped
1 tablespoon toasted sesame oil

Place the sesame seeds in a heatproof and flameproof frying pan and lightly toast them under a medium hot grill until they are just golden. Watch them constantly as they can burn quite easily. Steam the broccoli for 5–10 minutes, until tender. In a serving dish, combine the cooked broccoli, toasted sesame seeds and the oil. Mix well and serve.

Variations
Fry the broccoli in the oil instead of steaming it, for a different taste and texture. Use corn oil instead of toasted sesame oil.

Rice Pilaf

2 tablespoons butter
50 g (2 oz) chopped onion
225 g (8 oz) rice
475 ml (16 fl oz) gluten-free beef, chicken or vegetable stock or water

½ teaspoon salt
handful of fresh parsley, chopped

Preheat the oven to 180°C/350°F/Gas 4. Combine all the ingredients, except the parsley, in a buttered casserole dish. Cover and bake in the preheated oven for 1 hour. Sprinkle the parsley over the rice and serve.

Variations
Add mushrooms or any other vegetable you like.

Coriander Potatoes

4–5 potatoes, peeled and sliced
1–2 tablespoons butter
1 teaspoon chopped fresh coriander

Fry the potato slices in the butter until they are golden brown. Add the coriander 5 minutes before the potatoes are done, mixing it in evenly.

Variations
Add any herbs you like. Use olive oil instead of butter. Substitute sweet potatoes for the potatoes.

DESSERTS

You can have desserts again! Try making your own and you may be pleasantly surprised at the results.

Carrot Cake

3 eggs, separated
120 ml (4 fl oz) maple syrup or honey
100 g (4 oz) carrots, grated

100 g (4 oz) soya flour
100 g (4 oz) almonds, finely ground
½ teaspoon ground cinnamon

Preheat the oven to 190°C/375°F/Gas 5 and grease a 20 cm (8 in) square baking tin. Mix the egg yolks and maple syrup or honey together until you have a thick paste. Add the carrots, soya flour, almonds and cinnamon, mixing them together unitl well combined. Whisk the egg whites until stiff, then fold them gently into the carrot mixture. Pour the mixture into the prepeared tin and bake in the preheated oven for 45 minutes. It is done when a skewer inserted into the centre comes out clean.

Apple Spice Cake

450 g (1 lb) rice flour
350 g (12 oz) caster sugar
1 teaspoon bicarbonate of soda
1 teaspoon ground cinnamon
½ teaspoon ground nutmeg
½ teaspoon salt
3 eggs
250 ml (8 fl oz) corn oil

1 tablespoon gluten-free vanilla
  essence
900 g (2 lbs) apples, peeled,
  cored and sliced
225 g (8 oz) raisins
225 g (8 oz) walnuts, chopped

Preheat the oven to 180°C/350°F/Gas 4 and grease a 20 cm (8 in) baking tin. Combine the flour, sugar, bicarbonate of soda, spices and salt. Blend the eggs, oil and vanilla essence into the flour mixture. Fold the apples, raisins and walnuts into the batter. Pour the mixture into the prepared tin and bake in the preheated oven for 50–60 minutes. It is done when a skewer inserted into the centre comes out clean.

Variations
Use pecans instead of walnuts. Serve with whipped cream on top.

Chocolate Chip Cookies

275 g (10 oz) butter
450 g (1 lb) brown sugar
4 eggs
1 teaspoon gluten-free vanilla
   essence
550 g (1¼ lbs) rice flour
50 g (2 oz) potato flour

1 tablespoon gluten-free
   baking powder
1 teaspoon bicarbonate of soda
350 g (12 oz) pack gluten-free
   chocolate chips
100 g (4 oz) pecans

Preheat the oven to 190°C/375°F/Gas 5 and grease a baking sheet. Cream the butter and sugar together. Add the eggs and vanilla essence and mix them in well. Combine the flours, baking powder and bicarbonate of soda and add to the creamed mixture. Stir in the chocolate chips and nuts. Drop teaspoonfuls of the mixture onto the prepared baking sheet and bake in the preheated oven for 11–13 minutes.

Variations
Substitute honey or maple syrup for the brown sugar. Use walnuts instead of pecans.

Scones

275 g (10 oz) gluten-free flour
1 teaspoon baking powder
75 g (3 oz) butter
65 g (2½ oz) caster sugar

2 eggs
85 ml (3 fl oz) milk
50 g (2 oz) currants

Preheat the oven to 200°C/400°F/Gas 6 and grease a baking sheet. Mix the flour and baking powder together. Cream the butter, sugar, eggs and milk. Mix the dry ingredients and currants into the creamed mixture to form a soft dough. Drop teaspoonfuls of the mixture onto the prepared baking sheet and bake in the preheated oven for 15–20 minutes.

Variations
Add 50 g (2 oz) nuts. Use honey instead of the sugar. Substitute soya milk for the milk.

Gluten-free Pudding

165 ml (5½ fl oz) water
550 g (1¼ lbs) any soft fruit
75 g (3 oz) raw rice

2 tablespoons honey
½ teaspoon gluten-free vanilla
essence

Preheat the oven to 170°C/325°F/Gas 3. Bring the water to the boil, then add the fruit. Cook until it is soft. Process the fruit in a blender or food processor until smooth, then sieve it, removing any seeds or skin. Set aside 550 g (1¼ lbs) of the sieved fruit. Combine the rice, honey and vanilla essence in a 30 cm (12 in) square baking tin. Pour the set aside fruit over the top, cover the tin with foil and bake in the preheated oven for about 30 minutes, until the pudding has set.

Variations
Use different fruits – apples and plums are nice. Serve topped with yogurt or cream. Use maple syrup instead of the honey.

What if you're not a cook?

While the advantages of experimenting with gluten-free recipes are clear, if you don't like to cook you may never have to. There are gluten-free products you can buy if you want to avoid cooking. However, the range of foods you will be able to eat broadens dramatically if you do cook. This does not have to mean labouring over a hot cooker all day, as I hope you will have seen from the quick and easy recipes here. Start by allocating one day a week as your day to cook a new gluten-free recipe. Once you do it, you'll be amazed how easy it is to get into the habit of cooking your own foods ... and how delicious it is, too, so, go on, give it a try!

8

Getting rid of those gluten-free blues

Overcoming depression

It is not surprising that some coeliacs fall into a depression when they're starting on their gluten-free diet as, for many, their diet has to change radically. The thought of having to read food labels and think about everything that enters your mouth can be overwhelming, especially when you're still recovering from all the physical damage done by coeliac disease. As so many people have never had the responsibility for their own health placed on them before, it seems like a huge burden at first to go on a gluten-free diet.

In order to heal completely, you must heal on physical, mental and emotional levels. Sticking with a gluten-free diet will help you heal physically, but you cannot ignore the mental and emotional effects of doing this. Falling into a depression need not be serious – it doesn't mean you have to run to a psychiatrist. There are many ways to deal with how all this affects you mentally and emotionally on your own and in your own way.

'Checking in', as it were, with your mental and emotional selves is a good way to measure how you're feeling about the diet. Whether you think you're depressed about going on a gluten-free diet or not, check in with yourself by asking the following questions in relation to your new diet.

- Am I angry?
- Do I feel helpless?
- Am I frightened?
- Am I filled with dread?

Be honest with yourself. Feeling one or all of these emotions does not mean you're any different from many other coeliacs. Changing to a gluten-free diet in a gluten-drenched world is difficult. Once you listen to your emotions, coping with the diet will become easier.

The key to feeling positive about being on the diet is to create positive images for yourself. To do this, on one side of a piece of paper write down five negative thoughts you have had about your gluten-free diet. Look at each thought and, on the opposite side, rewrite the same thought in a positive way. Your negative thought has now been turned into a positive one. Being able to adopt these positive thoughts wholeheartedly may take some time, so pick one positive thought every week and try to begin to think in this way. Keep your list with you at all times and look at it periodically to remind yourself how you can feel positive about the diet.

Feeling blue about being on a gluten-free diet is normal, but you have to get over it if you want to fully recover. Don't adopt a stiff upper lip attitude that you're 'fine' when in fact you're not. This serves no purpose. If you feel down, actively try to do things that make you feel positive about the diet. This could make a huge difference in your life.

Five ways to pick yourself up

The following exercises will help you heal your mind and body on many levels. Not every exercise may be right for you, but try one or two and see if your attitude changes from negative to positive. Alternatively, create your own ways of coping, maybe by meditating or reading books on healing, and stick to your healing regimen. The diet will be a lot easier to stick to once you've adopted some coping mechanisms.

Have fun with gluten-free foods

If you think gluten-free foods are boring, think again. The positive side is that some gluten-free foods will probably be ones you've never eaten before, so being on this diet will give you the opportunity to try new foods. To make it interesting, you could do any of the following.

- *Have a gluten-free baking contest* See who can cook the best gluten-free cake among your family or friends. Pick a day to present your cakes and do a taste test, presenting the winner with a small prize. This is a great way to help your friends and family to a greater awareness of what gluten-free foods are and lessen their fear of cooking for you. Just touching something gluten-free can get rid of the mystique around gluten-free food. It doesn't have to be a cake competition – breads or biscuits are also great foods to experiment with!
- *Get the whole family involved in finding gluten-free foods at the supermarket.* Who can find the most gluten-free items in your local supermarket? This is a great way for kids to become involved and aware of what a gluten-free diet is. Allocate one morning a month for gluten-free shopping and take the whole family (and any friends who are interested and wish to tag along).

Take your guidelines for a gluten-free diet and the Coeliac Society's food list, so you can check any items you're unsure about. Everyone will have to read lots of labels. It may take some organizing, but it's worth it.

- *Cook a new dish once a month* Trying to substitute gluten-free versions of the foods you used to eat often leads to disappointment. Try cooking new dishes instead, using the gluten-free recipes in Chapter 7 as a starting point. Start slowly and don't overwhelm yourself too much by trying lots of new dishes at once. If you keep most of your meals simple, then dazzle yourself every month with a special meal, you're more likely too enjoy it.
- *Read more about health, food and healing* Information is empowering. The more you know about the foods you're eating, and health in general, the more this will encourage you to continue on the diet. When your health starts improving, you'll know the diet makes sense. Until then, spur yourself on by reading inspiring books on health, food and healing. When you're feeling down, they can be a great way to pick yourself up.

Join a coeliac support group

The benefits of sharing your ups and downs and useful information on this diet with other coeliacs can be tremendous. Contact the Coeliac Society (see Useful addresses at the end of the book) to find out if there is a group in your area. Every group is different, some organize coeliac experts to come to share the most up-to-date information on the disease and diet. Others do this and also have social events, with food and conversation.

You could start your own coeliac group, with like-minded coeliacs who want to meet and discuss what it is like to be a coeliac. If you do this, it's a good idea to find a doctor who specializes in coeliac disease who would be willing to answer specific questions about the disease that may arise in your support group. You may be surprised how beneficial listening to other coeliacs' feelings about the disease can be in helping you put your feelings into perspective and spark a very positive attitude towards staying on a gluten-free diet. When you know you're not alone, it can be a lot easier to keep going with the diet.

If you don't like the idea of a group, you could find a support person who is either a coeliac or a good listener and cares about your health – a 'healing friend'. Someone who picks you up when you're feeling down, encourages you to stay on the diet and is prepared to allow you to change in whatever way you need to.

Surrounding yourself with positive people who accept your diet is a very important part of coping on a gluten-free diet. Of course, family will need time to adjust to your diet, but will usually be there for you. With friends, you will know who among them will be your healing friends when a bit of time passes and some of them will be more willing to listen to you and care about your special needs than others. If you want healing friends, they will show up – don't force the issue. By believing it will happen and being open enough to talk about your needs, healing friends will appear.

Begin a coeliac diary

A diary is an excellent way to 'check in' with your emotions. It's also a great way to identify any lingering food intolerances you may have if your health is not improving on a gluten-free diet.

You can start a *coeliac diary* to record all your ups and downs while following the diet. Try to make an entry in the diary every day, even if it's very brief. You don't have to just write in your diary, you could draw, write poetry or paste in interesting articles. By doing this, the diary will take on the flavour of who you are and can be used to look back at and encourage yourself on the days when you feel a gluten-free diet is just too tough to follow.

If you think your health isn't improving due to food intolerances, start a *food and mood diary*. To do this, record on one side of the paper everything you eat and what time you eat it. On the other side, right down any abnormal physical or emotional sensations that arise during the day and when they occurred. After one week of tracking the foods you eat, look back at your diary and see if there is any reason to suspect you are having a reaction to any particular food. If so, eliminate that food for two weeks and then slowly reintroduce it and see how you feel. Pay particular attention to foods people are typically allergic to, like lactose, soya, corn and sugar.

Exercise

The power of exercise to reduce stress and create a positive attitude has been observed by many people. The key is to do an exercise you like. This may sound obvious, but far too many people push themselves to go to the gym every day – lifting weights or taking aerobics classes – when they actually don't like what they're doing. Exercise like this is less beneficial to your overall health and mental attitude than is doing a sport you enjoy, when you will be happy.

Sport does not have to mean breaking into a heavy sweat – walking 20 minutes every other day is extremely beneficial, for example. If you don't think you have enough time to do that, then walk on weekends. Do what you can, but try to do something – you will feel the benefits very quickly.

Laugh

It's incredible how many people go through life not laughing. Oh, what they are missing! Making time to laugh can help you put your new diet in perspective. It can dissolve negative feelings and open you up to considering new ways of looking at life. Follow my Five Commandments for Laughter throughout the day, reminding you to laugh:

The Five Commandments for Laughter
1 Every time you begin to feel upset about the diet, laugh.
2 Make a commitment to laugh for ten minutes every day.
3 Put coloured stickers around the house and every time you notice one, laugh.
4 Watch comedy shows.
5 Be around people who make you laugh.

A new beginning

This diet is the beginning of new eating habits for you and, naturally, it will present many challenges along the way. You don't have to be a hermit, disappearing from family and friends. A positive attitude will get you through a lot – use it and you will adhere to the diet and watch your health improve day by day. Just keep thinking, 'I am on the road to good health as long as I stick to a gluten-free diet'.

Always take time to evaluate how you're feeling, both physically and mentally. Think of this like your regular check-up, not replacing a visit to the doctor, which you must do if you're feeling really sick, but a way of getting to know your body better and taking care of yourself. Hopefully, as you see your health improving, this will encourage you not to cheat.

Every day you take a positive step, so will your health.

Appendix I: Coeliac disease on the Internet

Information is literally at your fingertips when you explore the Internet, and there is a wealth of information about coeliac disease. Much of it comes from the United States (where they spell coeliac 'celiac').

With any information you get, though, it is important not to quickly adopt it as being valid without checking it first. Every day we are learning more about coeliac disease, but as the Internet is international, keep in mind that products and procedures often differ between countries. When in doubt about the validity of any information, it's best to check with the Coeliac Society to see what it says.

Here are some sites you might like to call up.

- Celiac Listserv at St John's University is an open, unmoderated 'discussion list', accessed via e-mail, for those interested in coeliac disease. The discussions include the latest scientific research, information on what food is gluten-free and what is not, 'how to cope' issues, the connection between autism and coeliac disease, and gluten-free recipes. Almost everyone contributing to the list is a coeliac and it has members from all over the world, although the majority are American. The goal of the list is to act as a support group and information exchange forum on coeliac disease. To subscribe to the list, send an Internet e-mail message to 'LISTSERV@SJUVM.STJOHNS.EDU' and put in the body of the message 'SUBSCRIBE CELIAC', then your first and last name. For example, 'SUBSCRIBE CELIAC John Smith'. Do not write anything else in the body of the message, just send it like that. You will receive information about the list through e-mail. The Celiac Listserv also has a list for coeliac children and their parents called 'CEL-KIDS'. To subscribe, send an Internet e-mail to the same address as above, but, this time, in the body of the message write 'CEL-KIDS' and then your first and last name.
- For a comprehensive collection of coeliac-related sites on the worldwide web, have a look at Don Wiss' site at http://www.panix.com/~donwiss/
- To learn more about lactose intolerance Don Wiss also has another useful site at http://www.panix.com/~nomilk/

- For nutritional advice for coeliacs from the Vegetarian Society see http://www.veg.org/veg/Orgs/VegSocUK/Info/gluten.html
- A useful site for information on coeliac disease and a gluten-free diet is at http://www.demon.co.uk/webguides/nutrition/diets/glutenfree/index.html
- The Celiac Sprue Association of the United States of America (CSA/USA) has a homepage at http://members.aol.com/celiacusa/celiac.htm

Bibliography

Colbin, Annemarie, *Food and Healing*, Ballantine, 1986

Greer, Rita, *Gluten-free Cooking*, Thorsons, 1995

Hills, Hilda Cherry, *Good Food, Gluten-free*, Keats Publishing, New Canaan, Connecticut, 1976

Rosenvold, Lloyd, *Can a Gluten-free Diet Help? How?*, Keats Publishing, New Canaan, Connecticut, 1992

Turner, Kristina, *The Self-healing Cookbook*, Earthtones Press, 1987

Useful addresses and coeliac organizations around the world

The Coeliac Society
PO Box 200
High Wycombe
Buckinghamshire HP11 2HY

The Society is a trust set up for coeliacs in the UK. It provides information for coeliacs on the disease and coeliac support groups throughout the UK. Its bi-annual food list and magazine, *The Crossed Grain*, are available to all British coeliacs. Joining The Coeliac Society is the best way to keep informed on all aspects of coeliac disease, indeed, a hotline number is available for members to call for updates on their food list. Whenever you write to the Society and need a response, please enclose a SAE to help defray its operating costs.

The Gluten Free Pantry, Inc.
PO Box 840
Glastonbury, CT 06033, USA
Fax: 1 860 633 6853
e-mail: 72652.16@COMPUSERVE.COM

This company sells gluten-free products by mail order. It was created by a professional chef who is on a gluten-free diet.

Monastery of Poor Clares Colettines
Mossley Hill
Liverpool L18 3ES
or
The Carmelite Monastery of the Holy Ghost
Helenske Road
Dumbarton
G82 4AN

These two monasteries can provide you with gluten-free holy communion wafers, baked under the approval of the Archbishop of Liverpool.

Camp Sleath
Vashon Island
Washington State, USA
Tel: 1 206 463 3174

This camp provides a one-week session every summer where gluten-free meals are available for coeliac children. Other special diets can also be accommodated. The children attend all the normal activities – crafts, water sports and overnight camp-outs – but are served gluten-free meals, supervised by the Gluten Intolerance Group of North America (GIG). Call Camp Sleath or write to the GIG for details.

Suma Wholefoods
Dean Clough
Halifax HX3 5AN

This company can supply a small grain mill for grinding grains and pulses.

Trufree Foods Dept
225 Putney Bridge Road
London SW15 2PY

A vendor of gluten-free foods.

Virani Food Products Limited
Stewarts Road
Finedon Industrial Estate
Wellingborough
Northamptonshire NN8 4RJ

Another source of gluten-free foods.

Coeliac organizations around the world

ARGENTINA

Asistencia al Celiaco de la Argentina
Casila de Correo 5555
1000 Buenos Aires
Republica Argentina
Telex: 17354 Inserar
Fax: 541 331 3863

Asociacion Celiaco Argentina
Sede Central
Calle 2 No 1578, e/64 y 65
i900 La Plata
Buenos Aires
Republica Argentina
Tel: 54 21 31320/31030
Fax: 54 21 210288/30907

Asociacion Pro Ayuda Al Celiaco
Personeria Juridica 212 'A'
CC567 – Coreo Central – 5000
Cba
Cordoba
Republica Argentina

AUSTRALIA

The Coeliac Society of New South Wales
PO Box 271
Wahroonga 2076
New South Wales, Australia
Tel: 612 498 2593

The Coeliac Society of South Australia
106A Hampstead Road
Broadview 5083
South Australia, Australia
Tel: 61 8 266 3899

The Coeliac Society of Western Australia
PO Box 219
Mount Lawley 6050
Western Australia, Australia
Tel: 61 9 337 3504

The Queensland Coeliac Society
PO Box 530
Indooroopilly 4068
Queensland, Australia
Tel: 61 7 378 5747

The Victorian Coeliac Society
PO Box 22
Chadstone Centre 3148
Victoria, Australia
Tel: 61 3 772 7086

Victoria's Branch of the Coeliac Society in Tasmania
7 Bonar Place
Glenorchy
Tasmania 7010, Australia
Tel: 002 721024

AUSTRIA

Österreichische Arbeitsgemeinschaft Zoliakie
Anton-Baumgartner-Strasse 44/C5/2302
A-1232 Wien, Austria
Tel: 43 1 6708523

BELGIUM

SBMC-BCV
International Contacts
A20 Avenue L. Bertrand 100
B-1030 Brussels, Belgium
Tel: 32 2 216 8347
Fax: 32 216 8347

Vlaamse Coeliakievereniging
Ter Weibrock 29
L-9880 Aalter, Belgium
Tel: 32 1 74 28 45

BULGARIA

Bulgarian Coeliac Society
Pl. Slavieikov 9
Sofia 1000, Bulgaria

CANADA

Canadian Celiac Association
6519B Mississauga Road
Mississauga, ON L5N 1A6
Canada
Tel: 905 567 7195
  (In Canada: 800 363 7296)
Fax/answering machine: 905 567 0710

Fondation Quebecoise de la Maladie Coeliaque
(Quebec celiac foundation)
5115 Trans-Island, office #236
Montreal (Quebec)
Canada H3W 2Z9
Tel: 514 484 0454
Fax: 514 484 1320

DENMARK

Dansk Coliaki Forening
Bellisvej 31
DK-3650 Olstykke, Denmark
Tel: 45 4217 4664
(In summer: 45 9733 8345)

EGYPT

World Health Organisation
Dr M. H. Wahdan
PO Box 1517
Alexandria 21511, Egypt

ESTONIA

Tartu University
Professor V. Salupere
International Medical Clinic
Ulikooli 18
Tartu EE 2400, Estonia

FINLAND

The Finnish Coeliac Society
Mustanlahdenkatu 10
SF-33210 Tampere, Finland
Tel/fax: +358 31 2140 402

FRANCE

Association Française des Intolerants au Gluten
89 Rue du Faubourg Saint Antoine
F-75011 Paris, France
Tel: 33 1 43 47 0447

GERMANY

Deutsche Zoliakie-Gesellschaft
Filderhaupstrasse 61
Stuttgart 70, Germany
Tel: 33 711 454514
Fax: 49 711 4567817

GREECE

Hellenic Coeliac Society
125 Ippokratous Street
GR-Athens 114 72, Greece
Tel: 30 136 14 366
   or: 30 1 46 18 081

HUNGARY

Mrs Tunde Koltai
Liszterzekenyek Erdekkpviseletenek
Orszagos Egyesulete
Palanta U. 11
H-1025 Budapest, Hungary
Tel: 36 1 202 7396 and 6892
  or: 36 1 135 1278
Fax: 36 1 155 9816

ICELAND

Samtok Folks med Glutenopol
Logafold 15
IS-112 Reykjavik, Iceland
Tel: 354 675064
Fax: 354 603350

IRELAND

The Coeliac Society of Ireland
Carmichael House
4 North Brunswick Street
Dublin 4, Ireland
Tel: 353 1 31478

ISRAEL

The Israel Coeliac Society
Rehov Rabinowitz 9
ISR-96549 Jerusalem, Israel
Tel: 972 2 412635

ITALY

Associazione Famiglie Bambini Celiachi
Via Masia 21
I-40138 Bologna, Italy
Tel: 39 51 391980

Associazione Italiana Celiachi
Via S. Senatore 2
20122 Milano, Italy
Via Picotti 22
56124 Pisa, Italy
Tel/fax: +39 50 580939

MALTA

Coeliac Association
Mrs Mary Rose Caruana
'Lumet'
Upper Gardens
St Julians STJ 05, Malta
Tel: 35 370778

THE NETHERLANDS

Nederlandse Coeliakie Vereniging
Deimos 5
NL-3402 JG Ijsselstein, The Netherlands

NEW ZEALAND

Coeliac Society of New Zealand
18 Rutherford Terrace
Meadowbank
Auckland 5, New Zealand

NORWAY

Norsk Coliaki Forening
Prinsens Gate 6.5. etg.
N-0152 Oslo, Norway
Tel: 47 22 42 60 01
Fax: 47 22 42 60 04

POLAND

TPD
Magdalena Loska
U1. Jasna 24/26
PL-00-950 Warszawa, Poland
Tel: 48 22 27 78 44

PORTUGAL

Clube dos Coliacos
Pedietria Hospital Santa Maria
P-1600 Lisboa, Portugal
Tel: 351 749327

Portuguese Coeliac Association
Associacao Portuguesa dos Doentes com Intolerancia ao Gluten –
Clube dos Celiacos
Apartado 41005
1500 Lisboa Codex
Portugal

ROMANIA
Aglutena
Karin Kober
Sdr. Avram Ianca nr 24
2400 Sibiu, Romania
Tel: 417622
   or: 433050, extension 268

SLOVENIA

Slovensko Drustvo za Celiakijo
Ljubljanska 5
62000 Maribor, Slovenia

SOUTH AFRICA

Coeliac Society of South Africa
91 Third Avenue
Percelia 2192
Johannesburg, South Africa
Tel: 27 440 3431

SPAIN

ACE Delegacion Comtabria
Emmique Cueto
Apdo. Correos 291
E-39080 Santander, Spain
Tel: 34 33 63 85

ACM Associacion de Celiacos de Madrid
C/Pozas, 4-Local
E-28004-Madrid, Spain
Tel: 34 1 523 04 94

EZE Associacion Celiaca de Euzkadi
Somera. 3 – 30-Dpto 2
E-48005 Bilbao, Spain
Tel: 34 4 416 94 80

SMAP Celiacs de Catalunya
Madilde Torralba
Ronda Universidad No. 21–80-F
E-08007 Barcelona, Spain
Tel: 34 317 72 00, extension 98

SWEDEN

Svenska Celiakiforbundet
Box 9040
S-102 71 Stockholm, Sweden
Tel: 46 669 86 72
Fax: 46 668 74 05

SWITZERLAND

Associacion Romande dela Coeliakie
2 Avenue Agassiz
CH-1001 Lausanne, Switzerland
Tel: 021 319 71 11
Fax: 021 319 79 10

Gruppo della Svizzera Italiana degli Interessati al Problema della Celiachia
Fam. E + S Pedrazzoli
Contrada Isolabella 1, Pedevilla
Ch-6512 Giubiasco, Switzerland
Tel: 41 92 27 34 54

Schweizerische Interessengemeinschaft für Zoliakie
Schaulistrasse 4
CH-4142 Munchenstein, Switzerland
Tel: 41 61 46 21 87

UNITED KINGDOM

The Coeliac Society
PO Box 200
High Wycombe
Buckinghamshire HP11 2HY

UNITED STATES

Celiac Disease Foundation
13251 Ventura Boulevard, Suite 3
Studio City, CA 91604–1838, USA
Tel: 818 990 Celiac
  or: 818 990 2354
Celiac Sprue Association
PO Box 31700
Omaha, NE 68131–0700, USA
Tel: 402 558 0600

Gluten Intolerance Group of North America (GIG)
PO Box 23053
Seattle, WA 98102, USA
Tel: 206 325 6980

The Celiac ActionLine
Michael Jones
12733 Newfield Drive
Orlando, FL 32837
Tel: 407 856 3754

Index

Recipes